D0866160

# THE ROLE OF LEADERSHIP IN OCCUPATIONAL STRESS

# RESEARCH IN OCCUPATIONAL STRESS AND WELL BEING

Series Editors: Pamela L. Perrewé,
Jonathon R. B. Halbesleben
and Christopher C. Rosen

Recent Volumes:

RESEARCH IN OCCUPATIONAL STRESS AND
WELL BEING    VOLUME 14

# THE ROLE OF LEADERSHIP IN OCCUPATIONAL STRESS

## GUEST EDITORS

### WILLIAM A. GENTRY
*Center for Creative Leadership, Greensboro, NC, USA*

### CATHLEEN CLERKIN
*Center for Creative Leadership, Greensboro, NC, USA*

## SERIES EDITORS

### PAMELA L. PERREWÉ
*Florida State University, Tallahassee, FL, USA*

### JONATHON R. B. HALBESLEBEN
*University of Alabama, Tuscaloosa, AL, USA*

### CHRISTOPHER C. ROSEN
*University of Arkansas, Fayetteville, AR, USA*

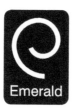

United Kingdom – North America – Japan
India – Malaysia – China

Emerald Group Publishing Limited
Howard House, Wagon Lane, Bingley BD16 1WA, UK

First edition 2016

Copyright © 2016 Emerald Group Publishing Limited

**Reprints and permissions service**
Contact: permissions@emeraldinsight.com

No part of this book may be reproduced, stored in a retrieval system, transmitted in any form or by any means electronic, mechanical, photocopying, recording or otherwise without either the prior written permission of the publisher or a licence permitting restricted copying issued in the UK by The Copyright Licensing Agency and in the USA by The Copyright Clearance Center. Any opinions expressed in the chapters are those of the authors. Whilst Emerald makes every effort to ensure the quality and accuracy of its content, Emerald makes no representation implied or otherwise, as to the chapters' suitability and application and disclaims any warranties, express or implied, to their use.

**British Library Cataloguing in Publication Data**
A catalogue record for this book is available from the British Library

ISBN: 978-1-78635-062-6
ISSN: 1479-3555 (Series)

ISOQAR certified
Management System,
awarded to Emerald
for adherence to
Environmental
standard
ISO 14001:2004.

Certificate Number 1985
ISO 14001

INVESTOR IN PEOPLE

# CONTENTS

# LIST OF CONTRIBUTORS

| | |
|---|---|
| *Melissa K. Carsten* | Department of Management and Marketing, College of Business Administration, Winthrop University, Rock Hill, SC, USA |
| *Rachel Clapp-Smith* | College of Business, Purdue University Northwest, Hammond, IN, USA |
| *Malissa A. Clark* | Department of Psychology, University of Georgia, Athens, GA, USA |
| *Cathleen Clerkin* | Center for Creative Leadership, Greensboro, NC, USA |
| *Kristin L. Cullen-Lester* | Center for Creative Leadership, Greensboro, NC, USA |
| *Jennifer K. Dimoff* | Department of Psychology, Saint Mary's University, Halifax, NS, Canada |
| *William A. Gentry* | Center for Creative Leadership, Greensboro, NC, USA |
| *Alexandra Gerbasi* | Surrey Business School, University of Surrey, Guildford, Surrey, UK |
| *Tracy L. Griggs* | Department of Management and Marketing, College of Business Administration, Winthrop University, Rock Hill, SC, USA |
| *Jonathon R. B. Halbesleben* | Department of Management, Culverhouse College of Commerce, University of Alabama, Tuscaloosa, AL, USA |
| *Michelle M. Hammond* | Kemmy Business School, University of Limerick, Limerick, Ireland |
| *P. D. Harms* | Department of Management, University of Alabama, Tuscaloosa, AL, USA |

| | |
|---|---|
| *E. Kevin Kelloway* | Department of Psychology, Saint Mary's University, Halifax, NS, Canada |
| *Gretchen Vogelgesang Lester* | Lucas College of Business, San Jose State University, San Jose, CA, USA |
| *Jesse S. Michel* | Department of Psychology, Auburn University, Auburn, AL, USA |
| *Michael E. Palanski* | Saunders College of Business, Rochester Institute of Technology, Rochester, NY, USA |
| *Pamela L. Perrewé* | College of Business, Florida State University, Tallahassee, FL, USA |
| *Christopher C. Rosen* | Department of Management, Sam M. Walton College of Business, University of Arkansas, Fayetteville, AR, USA |
| *Marian N. Ruderman* | Center for Creative Leadership, Greensboro, NC, USA |
| *Seth M. Spain* | School of Management, Binghamton University, New York, NY, USA |
| *Gregory W. Stevens* | Globoforce, Southborough, MA, USA |
| *Mary Uhl-Bien* | Department of Management, Entrepreneurship, and Leadership, Neeley School of Business, Texas Christian University, Fort Worth, TX, USA |
| *Sean White* | Grenoble Ecole de Management, Grenoble, France |
| *Dustin Wood* | Department of Management, University of Alabama, Tuscaloosa, AL, USA |
| *Lauren Zimmerman* | Department of Psychology, University of Georgia, Athens, GA, USA |

# EDITORIAL ADVISORY BOARD

Terry Beehr
*University of Central Michigan,*
*Department of Psychology, USA*

Chu-Hsiang (Daisy) Chang
*Michigan State University,*
*Department of Psychology, USA*

Yitzhak Fried
*Texas Tech – Rawls College of*
*Business, USA*

Dan Ganster
*Colorado State University,*
*Department of*
*Management, USA*

Leslie Hammer
*Portland State University,*
*Department of Psychology, USA*

Russ Johnson
*Michigan State University,*
*Department of Management, USA*

John Kammeyer-Mueller
*University of Minnesota, USA*

E. Kevin Kelloway
*Saint Mary's University,*
*Department of Psychology,*
*Canada*

Jeff LePine
*Arizona State University,*
*Department of Management, USA*

Paul Levy
*University of Akron, Department of*
*Psychology, USA*

John Schaubroeck
*Michigan State University, School*
*of Management and Department of*
*Psychology, USA*

Norbert Semmer
*University of Bern, Department of*
*Psychology, Switzerland*

Sabine Sonnentag
*Department of Psychology,*
*University of Mannheim, Germany*

Paul Spector
*University of South Florida,*
*Department of Psychology, USA*

Lois Tetrick
*George Mason University,*
*Department of Psychology, USA*

Mo Wang
*University of Florida, Department*
*of Management, USA*

# OVERVIEW

For this volume of *Research in Occupational Stress and Well Being*, we have partnered with guest editors from the *Center for Creative Leadership* to assemble a collection of unique insights examining occupational health through a leadership lens. This volume consists of seven chapters, each focusing on a different aspect of leadership and the role that leaders may play in facilitating stress and well-being in the workplace.

The first two chapters examine how certain traits and behaviors of leaders can exacerbate occupational stress. In the chapter "Workaholism among Leaders: Implications for Their Own and Their Followers' Well-Being," Malissa A. Clark, Gregory W. Stevens, Jesse S. Michel, and Lauren Zimmerman explore the issue of workaholism, and the negative impact that workaholic leaders can have in the workplace. They introduce a conceptual model linking workaholism to both leaders' and followers' well-being through affective, cognitive, and behavioral pathways. In the chapter "Stress, Well-Being, and the Dark Side of Leadership", Seth M. Spain, P. D. Harms, and Dustin Wood examine the role of dark side personality characteristics in the workplace. Using a functionalist approach, the authors provide a concise review of dark side characteristics and discuss how such characteristics might facilitate leader emergence and produce stress experiences for their followers.

The next three chapters of this volume examine the importance of interpersonal relationships to occupational health and well-being. In the chapter "The Promise and Peril of Workplace Connections: Insights for Leaders about Workplace Networks and Well-Being", Kristin L. Cullen-Lester, Alexandra Gerbasi, and Sean White focus on workplace connections and the power of leaders' networks. They propose that leaders' social connections can impact well-being through providing access to resources (e.g., information, feedback, and support) and highlight four key aspects of networks that can influence well-being − centrality, structural holes, embeddedness, and negative ties. In the chapter "Do You Believe What I Believe? A Theoretical Model of Congruence in Follower Role Orientation and Its Effects on Manager and Subordinate Outcomes", Melissa K. Carsten, Mary Uhl-Bien, and Tracy L. Griggs draw on relational leadership theory to examine a key ingredient of leadership: followership. The authors introduce a theoretical model detailing how congruence, or incongruence, between leaders' and followers' "follower role orientation" (i.e., beliefs about how to enact a follower role) can create both good and bad stress through leader-member exchange (LMX). In the chapter "An Enrichment/ Impairment Perspective on Leading in Multiple Domains: The Impact on Leader/Follower Well-Being and Stress," Michael E. Palanski, Gretchen Vogelgesang Lester, Rachel Clapp-Smith, and Michelle M. Hammond put forth a model of "multi-domain leadership" (MDL) that examines how leaders' knowledge, skills and abilities may be applied across multiple domains of life, such as work, community, and family. They describe both short-term and long-term effects of engaging in MDL, including how it may impact stress levels, self-efficacy, and self-awareness of leaders, as well as those around them.

The final section of this volume includes two chapters focusing on how leaders can promote workplace well-being. In the chapter "Resource Utilization Model: Organizational Leaders as Resource Facilitators," Jennifer K. Dimoff and E. Kevin Kelloway discuss the fact that despite high rates of health-related issues, and high availability of benefits, most employees fail to use the resources that are accessible to them. The authors introduce a perspective called "resource utilization theory" (RUT) to explain why employees do not use resources to deal with existing stressors, and propose that leaders hold a key role in facilitating the utilization of resources. In the chapter "Holistic Leader Development: A Tool for Enhancing Leader Well-Being", Cathleen Clerkin and Marian N. Ruderman argue that leader development initiatives need to be expanded to include well-being. They introduce a holistic development framework that focuses on building the intrapersonal competencies needed by modern leaders, and suggest that leader development is an underleveraged way to promote healthier work environments.

Together, these chapters illustrate the vital roles that leaders play in promoting well-being — or stress — in the workplace. Given this, we urge researchers and practitioners of occupational health to include discussions of leadership in their future work, in order to advance the field and create sustainable organizational change. We hope you enjoy this volume of *Research in Occupational Stress and Well Being*.

# ACKNOWLEDGMENTS

I would like to thank our guest editors, William A. Gentry and Cathleen Clerkin for taking on the role of guest editors for this volume. They managed the process beautifully and I am sure our readers will find this volume on the role of leadership in occupational stress and well-being to be very interesting, timely, and well done.

I would also like to acknowledge the contributions and hard work of Jonathon R. B. Halbesleben as co-editor of the series for the past five volumes. Due to his increased administrative responsibilities, he will no longer be able to co-edit *Research in Occupational Stress and Well Being*. Christopher C. Rosen and I would like to thank Jonathon for helping to make this series stronger and more visible. Jonathon has been a pleasure with whom to work, and Chris and I will miss working with our friend. Our very best to you, Jonathon.

Pamela L. Perrewé
*Editor*

# WORKAHOLISM AMONG LEADERS: IMPLICATIONS FOR THEIR OWN AND THEIR FOLLOWERS' WELL-BEING

Malissa A. Clark, Gregory W. Stevens, Jesse S. Michel and Lauren Zimmerman

## ABSTRACT

*This chapter examines the role of leader workaholism in relation to their own and their followers' well-being. We begin with an overview of workaholism, along with a description of how workaholism may relate to typical leader behaviors. We propose a conceptual model linking the various components of workaholism to leaders' well-being and followers' well-being. In our model, we propose that leaders' workaholism can negatively influence their own well-being, and also their followers' well-being through interindividual crossover of affective, cognitive, and behavioral components of workaholism. Furthermore, the negative well-being outcomes experienced by the workaholic leader can also crossover to the followers through interindividual strain–strain crossover. Several*

The Role of Leadership in Occupational Stress
Research in Occupational Stress and Well Being, Volume 14, 1–31
Copyright © 2016 by Emerald Group Publishing Limited
All rights of reproduction in any form reserved
ISSN: 1479-3555/doi:10.1108/S1479-355520160000014001

*moderating factors of these relationships are discussed, as well as avenues for future research.*

**Keywords:** Workaholism; leadership; well-being; crossover

# INTRODUCTION

A multitude of evidence suggests that employees in the United States are working increasingly long hours, both in terms of annual hours worked (Murphy & Sauter, 2003; Schor, 2003) and hours worked per week (Brett & Stroh, 2003; Kuhn & Lozano, 2008). Data from countries outside the United States tell a similar story, especially in Asian and Eastern European countries, like Singapore, South Korea, Hong Kong, Poland, and Hungary where average annual working hours are higher than the United States (Organization and Economic Cooperation and Development, 2015). According to a study conducted by the International Labor Organization, Americans put in the equivalent of an extra 40-hour work week in 2000 compared to 1990 (Greenhause, 2001). Furthermore, more recent labor trends indicate that the average number of hours worked per week by Americans has steadily increased from 44.9 hours in 2005 and 2006 to 46.7 hours in 2013 and 2014 (Gallup, 2014). This trend toward ever-increasing work hours is only likely to be exacerbated with the growing expectation from organizations that employees use communication technology (including telephone calls, e-mails, and texting) for work purposes after work hours (Harris, Marett, & Harris, 2011).

How does this increased work time and organizational expectations for employees to be constantly "connected" to work via technology affect employees? A recent study found that managers, professionals, and executives who use smartphones for work report that they interact with work a staggering 13.5 hours every workday (Deal, 2015). This constant interaction with work has the potential for negative impacts on worker well-being. Research in the area of job stress has shown that when employees are able to psychologically detach from work during off-job time, this allows them to regulate their affect over the course of the work week, and this psychological detachment becomes even more crucial for employee well-being when the employees are highly engaged in their work (Sonnentag, Mojza, Binnewies, & Scholl, 2008). Reflecting these broader societal trends in increasing work hours (e.g., Kuhn & Lozano, 2008) and the idea that constant involvement with work with no respite can lead to negative outcomes (Sonnentag et al., 2008), the amount of attention to workaholism has steadily increased over the past couple of decades. Workaholism has been extensively covered in the popular press (Lavine, 2014; Singal, 2014; Stillman, 2014), indicating that the general public is just as concerned with employee overwork (or perhaps even more so) as academics. In fact, a recent *New York Times* piece highlighted several real-life examples of the dire consequences of extreme levels of work involvement in the investment banking field: professionals in their 20s who have reportedly died as a result of prolonged periods of intense working without rest (Cohan, 2015).

Despite the increased attention given to workaholism both in the popular press as well as in the academic literature, we know surprisingly little about the intersection of workaholism and leadership. For example, what are the potential well-being outcomes for a workaholic leader? What about his or her followers? In the current chapter, to explore these ideas we first provide an overview of the workaholism construct, its correlates, and outcomes. Next, we provide an introduction to some key leadership theories that may best inform our understanding of workaholic leaders. We then explore (1) well-being outcomes for the workaholic leader and the role of leaders' individual differences, and (2) well-being outcomes for followers of the workaholic leader, with a focus on specific leader-follower crossover mechanisms. The chapter concludes with recommendations for future research that can help advance our understanding of these concepts.

### Workaholism: Initial Overview

The term workaholism was first coined by psychologist and minister Oates (1971), who defined workaholism as "addiction to work, the compulsion or uncontrollable need to work incessantly" (p. 11). Since then, workaholism has been described in a variety of different ways: as an addiction to work (Ng, Sorensen, & Feldman, 2007; Porter, 2006; Robinson, 2000), a pathology (Fassel, 1990), a behavior pattern that persists across multiple organizational settings (Scott, Moore, & Miceli, 1997) and a syndrome comprised of high drive, high work involvement, and low work enjoyment (Aziz & Zickar, 2006). In an effort to reconcile these varied perspectives, in a previous paper we identified key commonalities across these definitions and used these to form a comprehensive definition of the construct. Specifically, we define workaholism as "an addiction to work that involves feeling compelled or driven to work because of internal pressures, having persistent and frequent thoughts about work when not working, and working beyond what is reasonably expected (as established by the requirements of the job or basic economic needs) despite potential negative consequences" (Clark, Michel, Zhdanova, Pui, & Baltes, 2014, p. 5).

Some have argued that workaholism is associated with positive outcomes such job satisfaction, experiencing a high level of eustress (pleasant stress) and high performance (Baruch, 2011). Baruch also posits that workaholics may serve as role models for other employees. Additionally, others have speculated that workaholism may lead to positive outcomes (e.g., job satisfaction, job performance) in the short-term but negative outcomes (e.g., poor health, relationship problems) in the long-term (Ng et al., 2007). However, the question of whether workaholism may be positive in the short-term but negative in the long-term has not yet been empirically examined. Cross-sectional research on workaholism and outcomes has overwhelmingly shown that workaholism is related to negative individual, work, and family outcomes (Andreassen, Hetland, Molde, & Pallesen, 2011; Brady, Vodanovich, & Rotunda, 2008; van Beek, Taris, & Schaufeli, 2011). Prior to discussing the intersection of leadership and workaholism, we begin with a brief description of the nomological network of workaholism, including how workaholism relates to other personality constructs, the difference between workaholism and work engagement, and relationships between workaholism and outcomes.

## Nomological Network of Workaholism

### Personality Correlates

The most commonly studied personality characteristics in relation to workaholism are achievement-oriented traits. Meta-analytic evidence shows perfectionism ($\rho = .46$) and Type A personality ($\rho = .32$) have fairly strong correlations with workaholism (Clark et al., 2014). Additionally, workaholism appears to have stronger relationships with maladaptive (e.g., when one perceives a high discrepancy between one's performance expectations and current performance), but not adaptive (e.g., possessing high standards and performance expectations of oneself) dimensions of perfectionism (Clark, Lelchook, & Taylor, 2010). Narcissism has also been shown to positively relate to workaholism (Andreassen, Ursin, Eriksen, & Pallesen, 2012; Clark et al., 2010). Of the Big Five personality traits, conscientiousness, extraversion, neuroticism, and openness are positively related to workaholism, and agreeableness is negatively related to workaholism (Andreassen, Hetland, & Pallesen, 2010; Burke, Matthiesen, & Pallesen, 2006; Clark et al., 2010). These relationships are relatively weak, however, and there is a good deal of variability across studies. Meta-analytic evidence shows workaholism is positively related to trait negative affect ($\rho$ = .25), while it is not significantly related to trait positive affect ($\rho$ = −.02; Clark et al., 2014).

*Distinguishing Workaholism from Work Engagement*
Workaholism can be distinguished from the construct of work engagement, which refers to "a positive, fulfilling, work-related state of mind that is characterized by vigor, dedication, and absorption" (Schaufeli, Salanova, González-Romá, & Bakker, 2002). Undoubtedly, the behaviors of workaholics and engaged workers appear similar because in both cases these individuals often work harder and longer than other individuals. However, research suggests one key difference between workaholism and work engagement is the motivations underlying these behaviors. Whereas engaged workers are driven to work because they find it intrinsically pleasurable, workaholics are driven to work because they feel an inner compulsion to work — feelings that they "should" be working (Graves, Ruderman, Ohlott, & Weber, 2012). Several studies have found support for the idea that workaholism and work engagement are related to different motivational underpinnings (Clark, Hunter, Beiler-May, & Carlson, 2015; van Beek, Hu, Schaufeli, Taris, & Schreurs, 2012; van Beek, Taris, Schaufeli, & Brenninkmeijer, 2014). A second key difference is that work engagement, unlike workaholism, is primarily linked with positive outcomes such as increased job satisfaction, task and contextual performance. Furthermore, workaholism and work engagement often show differential relationships with certain personality traits such as positive affect (Christian, Garza, & Slaughter, 2011; Clark et al., 2014).

*Outcomes of Workaholism*
As will be discussed in more detail later in the chapter, a cumulative body of research supports the idea that workaholism is associated with negative outcomes for the individual, for the workaholic's family, and even for the organization. In terms of individual outcomes, workaholics have lower life satisfaction (Andreassen et al., 2011), poor physical and mental health, and greater burnout (Schaufeli, Taris, & Bakker, 2008). Workaholics also experience negative family outcomes such as greater work−life conflict

(Andreassen, Hetland, & Pallesen, 2013). Regarding organizational out-comes, unlike work engagement (which as noted previously has been shown to positively relate to task performance) workaholism is typically unrelated to work performance (Clark et al., 2014). This may suggest that even though workaholics may spend more time thinking about and physically engaging in work than the average worker, this may not translate into better work performance. Additionally, workaholics experience greater job stress (Burke, 2001), are more likely to engage in counterproductive work behaviors (Balducci, Cecchin, Fraccaroli, & Schaufeli, 2012), and have lower job satisfaction (Andreassen et al., 2011) than nonworkaholics.

## WORKAHOLISM AND LEADERSHIP: AN INITIAL FOUNDATION

Despite interest in the workaholic leader among practitioners (e.g., Meinert, 2014), there is a relative dearth of theoretical or empirical litera-ture connecting these two areas of research. Recent research has pointed to the utility of considering the dual impact of leadership traits and behaviors, particularly as those behaviors mediate the relationship between leader traits and outcomes (DeRue, Nahrgang, Wellman, & Humphrey, 2011). Although a number of behaviors have been proposed in the leadership literature, the majority can be distilled down to several key domains: task-oriented, relational-oriented, change-oriented, and passive behaviors (DeRue et al., 2011; McCauley, 2004). These domains offer a useful frame-work for understanding the ways in which workaholism may impact the functions and responsibilities of the leader role.

### Task-Oriented Behaviors

These types of behaviors are focused on a range of task processes, such as defining roles, coordination, determining standards of task performance, and so forth. Popular leadership theories that fall into this domain include initiating structure (Judge, Piccolo, & Ilies, 2004), forms of transactional leadership (Bass & Avolio, 1995), and active management-by-exception (MBE; Avolio, Bass, & Jung, 1999). Workaholic leaders may find more congruence within this domain of leadership behaviors, given the amount of time and focus they devote to their own work and by extension, the work of those underneath them. Furthermore, workaholic leaders may be prone to establishing and clarifying roles for accomplishing tasks, as well as monitoring the ongoing completion of those tasks. To the extent that such behaviors also require the leader to take on responsibility for the completion of a set of tasks, the workaholic leader may experience greater fit within these types of responsibilities.

## Relational-Oriented Behaviors

This set of behaviors includes those that are primarily focused on building relationships among team members and encouraging those members to perform on behalf of the group. Leadership theories that address relational aspects of leadership fall into this domain, including aspects of transformational leadership (Bass, 1999), consideration (Judge et al., 2004), and a range of approaches focused on empowering followers (e.g., Chen, Kirkman, Kanfer, Allen, & Rosen, 2007) and encouraging participative approaches (e.g., Huang, Iun, Liu, & Gong, 2010; Somech, 2003). Workaholic leaders may have difficulty focusing on the relational aspects of work, given their proclivity toward completing tasks. The amount of time that is needed to devote toward mentoring subordinates or developing teams may only be seen as time away from the actual work that needs to be accomplished. Moreover, the sense of anxiety and guilt surrounding not ever having done enough work may work to the detriment of subordinates seeking recognition for their contributions to the team.

## Change-Oriented Behaviors

The third broad set of behaviors includes those focused on responding to and driving change within groups. Broadly, leaders exhibiting change behaviors are focused on creating and communicating a shared vision, as well as encouraging creative or innovative thinking and risk-taking. Aspects of transformational leadership, including inspirational motivation and intellectual stimulation (Bass, 1999; Bono & Judge, 2004), fall into this set of behaviors. This set of behaviors may present particular challenges to the workaholic leader, primarily in terms of that leader's ability to effectively delegate work, to deal with fast-paced changes in light of correlations with rigid beliefs (Van Wijhe, Peeters, & Schaufeli, 2014), and empowering other employees to adopt their own flexible work styles.

*Passive-Oriented Behaviors*

The final set of leader behaviors reflects an absence of the typical types of behaviors that one might expect of his or her leader, either through inaction or only exhibiting behaviors when challenges or problems develop. Common examples of these types of behaviors include laissez-faire leadership and passive management-by-exception (Avolio et al., 1999). Workaholics who may be focused primarily on their own work compulsions or otherwise put themselves first (De Cremer & Van Dijk, 2005) rather than the work of the groups they lead may be more likely to engage in passive leadership behaviors that allow them to ignore those leadership behaviors that, on the face, do not support their ability to get work done (e.g., mentoring, supporting, networking). As such, workaholic leaders may be more likely to avoid leadership tasks until they begin to interfere with the ability to get work done.

Although the preceding typology of leadership behaviors has been well established within the literature (cf. McCauley, 2004), very little if any attention has been paid to the potential ways in which workaholism may be expressed across these different domains and its impact on relevant outcomes. The review is nevertheless presented in order to more fully establish the context in which workaholic leaders and their relationships with followers are situated. This context provides the background against which our conceptual model is established, describing the ways in which the components of workaholism influence the leader's own well-being outcomes, woven across relational and task-focused domains, as well as addressing approach (i.e., change-oriented) versus avoidant (i.e., passive-oriented) aspects. The foundation of leadership behaviors also influences the way in which the leader's workaholism relates to follower well-being, through various crossover mechanisms that similarly address cognitive, affective, and behavioral aspects of tasks, relationships, and change.

# A CONCEPTUAL MODEL LINKING CORE WORKAHOLISM DIMENSIONS TO LEADER AND FOLLOWER WELL-BEING OUTCOMES

Our conceptual model (illustrated in Fig. 1) draws from recent developments in the leadership literature toward more integrative frameworks (Avolio, 2007; DeRue et al., 2011) to explain the relationships between

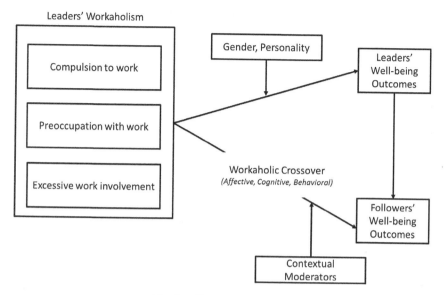

*Fig. 1.* Conceptual Model.

workaholic leadership and well-being outcomes for leaders and followers alike. Across the first two sections, we expand upon the core features of workaholism (i.e., compulsion to work, preoccupation with work, and excessive work involvement) and capture the ways in which they may influence well-being outcomes for workaholic leaders. We also consider the potential moderating effects of other traits that have historically been associated with leadership research (e.g., demographics, personality; DeRue et al., 2011).

Next, we consider the impact that workaholism may have on follower well-being. We argue that crossover theory (Westman, 2001, 2011) may suggest two distinct pathways to be influential in these relationships. First, the expression of leaders' workaholism itself may be transmitted to followers and impact their well-being, primarily through affective, cognitive, and behavioral aspects of workaholism (termed workaholic crossover). Second, leaders' negative well-being may itself directly influence follower well-being, through more traditional strain–strain crossover processes. We argue that these crossover effects may be moderated by the context in which the leader–follower relationships take place.

## The Workaholic Leader

Incorporating our multidimensional definition of workaholism, we propose that each of the core dimensions of workaholism (i.e., feelings of compulsion to work, cognitive preoccupation with work, and excessive involvement in work) should be considered when examining the relationship between workaholism and well-being outcomes.

### Compulsion to Work

The first core dimension of workaholism is that workaholics are driven to work because of an internal compulsion or need to work that cannot be resisted or controlled (Oates, 1971; Schaufeli, Taris, & Bakker, 2008; Spence & Robbins, 1992). Essentially, workaholics often feel compelled to work or obligated to work because of an inner feeling that one "should" be engaging in this behavior. Furthermore, this internal need or compulsion to work is said to stem from introjected motivation (Graves et al., 2012). According to self-determination theory, introjected motivation is when individuals experience inner demands to engage in behaviors and suffer ego deficits when they do not meet those demands (Deci & Ryan, 1985). In the case of workaholics, the ego deficits come in the form of feelings of guilt or anxiety when they are not working (Scott et al., 1997; Spence & Robbins, 1992). Interestingly, recent research has shown that workaholics not only are more likely to experience negative emotions while they are not at work, but they also are more likely to experience negative emotions and less likely to experience positive emotions at work (Clark, Michel, Stevens, Howell, & Scruggs, 2014). Given widespread evidence of the deleterious effects of negative moods and emotions (Elfenbein, 2007), feelings of guilt or anxiety experienced by workaholics due to their inner compulsion are likely to decrease not only their own well-being, but also their followers' well-being through the process of emotional contagion (or the "catching" of negative emotions; Barsade, 2002).

### Cognitive Preoccupation with Work

The second core dimension of workaholism is that the workaholic constantly thinks about work when they are not working and have a very difficult time disengaging from work (Schaufeli, Taris, & Bakker, 2008; Scott et al., 1997; Spence & Robbins, 1992). This cognitive preoccupation is something that is not easily suppressed or controlled (Smith & Seymour, 2004). Based on the idea that individuals have a finite amount of cognitive resources (i.e., resource drain theory; Edwards & Rothbard, 2000), persistent and uncontrollable thoughts about work may interfere with an individual's ability to devote their attention to nonwork demands or tasks. Indeed, preoccupation with work while not at work has been found to relate to lower life satisfaction and greater work–nonwork conflict (Ezzedeen & Swiercz, 2007).

*Excessive Involvement in Work*
The third dimension of workaholism concerns the workaholic's actual involvement with work. Not surprisingly, workaholics tend to work longer and harder than others, even when it is not required of them and even if it goes beyond what is reasonably expected of them (Robinson, 1998; Schaufeli, Taris, & Bakker, 2008; Scott et al., 1997). Because of this excessive work involvement, workaholics may miss family events, work on the weekends or weeknights, or consistently bring work home with them. The behavioral dimension of workaholism is so central to the construct that some researchers use hours worked as an indicator of workaholism (Snir & Harpaz, 2012); although many others have pointed out that workaholism is more than simply excessive behavioral involvement (Schaufeli, Taris, & Bakker, 2008). As Machlowitz (1978) stated, "workaholics are better defined by their relationship to their work than by the number of hours they work" (p. 6). In support of the idea that workaholism is much more than simply hours spent working, meta-analytic evidence shows workaholism and hours worked per week are only moderately correlated ($\rho = .30$ based on data from 20 samples; Clark et al., 2014). Nonetheless, while it is not the only criterion for workaholism, excessive work involvement is an important feature of workaholism. Overall, each of the core components of workaholism needs to be considered when examining the relationship between leader workaholism and outcomes.

*Outcomes of Leaders' Workaholic Behaviors*

People in leadership roles are particularly likely to experience the affective, cognitive, and behavioral aspects of workaholism. Indeed, research has shown that the occupational classification of managerial status alone is related to workaholism (Clark et al., 2014). Additionally, people in leadership roles are likely to experience high levels of work role overload, time commitment to the job, and job involvement and centrality, which are all strongly related to the experience of workaholism (e.g., Schaufeli, Taris, & Van Rhenen, 2008; van Beek, Hu, Schaufeli et al., 2012). Though leaders are in positions to experience higher levels of workaholism, we argue that leaders experience similar well-being outcomes as other workaholics in the labor force. However, in addition to experiencing higher levels of workaholism, and subsequent negative well-being outcomes, certain leaders may experience stronger consequences contingent on a number of moderating variables. In this section we describe likely well-being outcomes for the workaholic leader based on previous empirical literature, followed by a focus on key potential moderators of the leaders' workaholism—outcomes relationships based on previous research and theoretical propositions.

Based on an emerging body of workaholism literature, the workaholic leader should experience a number of negative outcomes such as decreased satisfaction, physical health, and emotional/mental health, as well as increased stress, burnout, and work—life conflict. In this section we outline previous literature related to work, family, and individual outcomes. Specifically, we suggest that: (1) the work-related outcomes of job satisfaction, job stress, and job burnout; (2) the family-related outcomes of family satisfaction, and work—family conflict; and (3) the individual outcomes of life satisfaction, emotional/mental health, and physical health are key consequences of leaders' workaholism and workaholic behaviors.

*Work-Related Outcomes*
Though workaholics are generally compelled or driven to work because of internal pressures, and have persistent and frequent thoughts about work when not working, they do not necessarily experience higher levels of job satisfaction. In fact, workaholics generally experience lower levels of job satisfaction, which is commonly referred to as an affective attachment or reaction (pleasurable or positive emotional state) to one's job or job experiences (Spector, 1997). For example, a study by Andreassen and colleagues (2011) examining well-being and health in a cross-occupational sample (e.g., pharmaceutical, healthcare, TV station, HR-sector, university faculty) found workaholics experienced lower levels of job satisfaction ($r = -.33$ for driven to work). Though this sample did not focus on leaders, as little workaholism literature does, the sample adequacy is high given the sample was largely educated and representative of the general labor force. Similarly, several samples by Schaufeli, Bakker, van der Heijden, and Prins (2009b) examining burnout and well-being found similar effects between workaholism and job satisfaction among skilled professionals ($r = -.20$ to $-.29$ for working compulsively and working excessively).

Job stress has also been proposed as a meaningful and significant outcome of workaholic behavior (e.g., Clark et al., 2014). Job stress generally refers to work conditions leading to reactions of strain, such as negative arousal, psychological impairments, and physical symptoms (Kahn & Byosiere, 1992). A number of studies have consistently shown strong positive relationships between workaholism and job stress. For example, Burke (2001) found that job stress was strongly correlated ($r = .50$) to driven to work in a sample of MBA graduates, of which 80% placed themselves into middle-or senior-management levels. Similarly, in the classic workaholism study by Spence and Robbins (1992), the authors found very large effect sizes ($r = .64$ to .66) between job stress and driven to work in both male and female samples. In fact, these effect sizes are so large in magnitude, some would argue that they approximate construct overlap (e.g., it is commonly argued that observed values approaching or exceeding $r = .70$ indicates a single construct, Berry, Ones, & Sackett, 2007).

Finally, job burnout has been an outcome of interest in the larger workaholism literature garnering significant research attention. Burnout is generally defined as a prolonged response to chronic emotional and interpersonal stressors on the job (Maslach, Schaufeli, & Leiter, 2001). In a study of telecom managers, Schaufeli, Taris, and Bakker (2008) found that workaholism, particularly being propelled by an inner drive, was related to the burnout dimensions of emotional exhaustion (depletion of one's emotional and physical resources), cynicism (excessive and negative detachment response), and inefficacy (lack of achievement, productivity, and feelings of incompetence). Additional primary studies across multiple job categories and industries have shown similar results (e.g., van Beek et al., 2011). Indeed, recent meta-analytic work by Clark et al. (2014) found that workaholism was related to higher levels of overall burnout ($\rho = .40$) as well as its elements (e.g., emotional exhaustion, $\rho = .42$).

*Family-Related Outcomes*
There has been a similar pattern of results for family-related outcomes of workaholism. For example, the literature suggests a general decrease in family satisfaction for workaholics. Similar to job satisfaction, family satisfaction is generally defined as an affective attachment or reaction (pleasurable or positive emotional state) to one's family or family experiences. A number of studies by Burke and colleagues (e.g., Burke & Fiksenbaum, 2009; Burke, 1999) have found small to moderate relationships ($r = -.10$ to $-.29$) between feeling driven to work/work addiction and family satisfaction. Additionally, many of these samples contain a large proportion of highly educated participants (e.g., all participants above Bachelor's degree) who were typically married with children, while one sample consisted of 88% practicing managers with MBA degrees. Additionally, research

examining family functioning in workaholics anonymous members has found strong negative relationships with family affective responsiveness and family affective involvement ($r = -.28$ and $-.25$), as well as other components of general family functioning (e.g., problem solving, communication; Robinson & Post, 1995).

The most frequently examined family-related outcome of workaholism has been the construct of work–family conflict, which is traditionally defined as a form of interrole conflict in which the work and family roles are mutually incompatible resulting in decreased work and family performance (Greenhaus & Beutell, 1985). Brady and colleagues (2008) examined the impact of workaholism on work–family conflict with a sample of Society for Human Resource Management (SHRM) members. Brady and colleagues found a strong positive relationship between overall workaholism and work–family conflict ($r = .47$). Additional researchers have found similar relationships across a variety of jobs/occupations (e.g., university employees, executives) and industries (e.g., education, healthcare, government agencies; Andreassen et al., 2013; Bakker, Demerouti, & Burke, 2009).

*Individual Outcomes*

A primary focus of the workaholism literature has been individual health and well-being outcomes. One area of this focus has been on the variables life satisfaction, life happiness, and general well-being. An empirical example is a longitudinal study by Peiperl and Jones (2001) which utilized a sample of managers and professionals with MBA degrees. Peiperl and Jones found that workaholism, operationalized as perceived time, effort, and balance of rewards, was related to a number of life satisfaction elements, including personal life outside work, family, standard of living, quality of life, balance of life in general. Similarly, Schaufeli, Bakker, Van der Heijden, and Prins (2009a) found that working compulsively and working excessively were moderate predictors of life satisfaction ($r = -.24$ to $-.32$) in a large sample from the healthcare industry, which is consistent with recent meta-analytic evidence suggesting uncorrected and corrected relationships around $r = -.25$ and $\rho = -.32$ (Clark et al., 2014).

A substantial proportion of the workaholism literature has also examined the individual outcomes of emotional/mental health and physical health, where emotional/mental health generally consist of interrelated constructs such as psychological strain, psychological distress, emotional well-being, and mental health, while physical health typically generally includes health complaints and psychosomatic symptoms. For physical health, both Graves et al. (2012) and Schaufeli, Taris, and Van Rhenen (2008) found small to moderate effect size magnitudes between workaholism and psychological strain/distress among managerial samples. Similarly, a number of managerial samples displayed comparable main effects (e.g., Bartczak & Ogińska-Bulik, 2012; Schaufeli, Taris, & Van Rhenen, 2008). Meanwhile, for physical health, specifically psychosomatic symptoms, Schaufeli et al. found moderate to large effect sizes ($r = .30$ to $.60$) for feelings of driven to work and working excessively. Again, these results seem to be stable across a large number of studies on health complaints and psychosomatic symptoms (e.g., Bartczak & Ogińska-Bulik, 2012; Taris, Geurts, Schaufeli, Blonk, & Lagerveld, 2008).

## Moderators of Leaders' Workaholism and Leaders' Well-Being Outcomes

In addition to the above workaholism main effects, we believe there may be moderating effects that will increase or decrease these leader workaholism–outcomes relationships. While there are certainly many characteristics that can play a role in leader workaholism-outcome relationships (e.g., a leader's level of work and family centrality), in the present chapter we focused on two characteristics that have traditionally been associated with leadership research: gender, and personality/individual differences.

### Gender

Although meta-analytic evidence suggests there are no main effect gender differences in workaholism (Clark et al., 2014), theories of gender role socialization and expectations (Eagly, 1987) suggest competing hypotheses regarding the extent to which male and female workaholic leaders may experience different negative outcomes. On the one hand, according to Blair-Loy's (2003) cultural schemas of work and family devotion, men's heavy investment in work is more socially acceptable than women's devotion to work because it is in line with the male as breadwinner stereotype. As men seek to attain this worker ideal, men may experience greater negative well-being outcomes. In support of this idea, meta-analytic evidence suggests samples with higher proportions of men exhibit a stronger relationship between workaholism and physical health outcomes than samples with higher proportions of women (Clark et al., 2014). On the other hand, these work and family devotion schemas (Blair-Loy, 2003) may suggest that workaholic women experience greater negative outcomes (e.g., burnout, work−family conflict) than workaholic men as their heavy investment in work conflicts with female gender role expectations to devote themselves solely to their family role. Thus, workaholic women's competing work and family demands and gender role expectations may lead them to experience greater negative well-being consequences than men workaholics. Future research is needed in this area, as we are not aware of any primary empirical studies examining the relationship between workaholism and well-being outcomes as moderated by gender.

*Personality and Individual Differences*
The importance of personality and individual differences for explaining a broad spectrum of attitudes and behaviors has received significant attention and support within the organizational literature (see Barrick & Mount, 2005; Hogan, 2005). Personality and individual differences represent mental structures and processes that influence a person's emotional and behavioral responses to their environment (i.e., characteristic patterns of behavior, thoughts, and feelings). Thus, personality and individual differences denote a predisposition or tendency to perceive and behave in a relatively consistent manner across time and situations (Hogan, 1991).

Several individual difference variables, such as trait negative affect (NA), perfectionism, and Type A personality, should moderate the leader workaholism and leader outcome relationship. Trait NA is defined as a general tendency to feel anxious, guilty, and upset (Watson & Clark, 1992); perfectionists tend to hold themselves to high personal standards, have a strong preference for order, and perceive a large discrepancy between their current and expected performance levels (Slaney, Rice, Mobley, Trippi, & Ashby, 2001); and Type A personality describes people who are generally aggressive, competitive, ambitious, impatience, and achievement striving (Bluen, Barling, & Burns, 1990; Edwards & Baglioni, 1991). Considering people high in trait NA have a predisposition to feelings of guilt and anxiety, and workaholics worry about work and feel guilty and anxious when not working (Ng et al., 2007; Scott et al., 1997), workaholics high in NA should experience even stronger negative outcomes of workaholism due to a general tendency to perceive and react in a consistent negative manner. Likewise, since perfectionists hold themselves to high standards, yet perceive their performance far from their ideal, perfectionists are more likely to be concerned with and react to their work behaviors than non-perfectionists. Finally, considering Type A people are competitive and ambitious, it makes sense that Type A personalities will have more extreme responses to workaholism than non-Type A personalities.

In all cases, we believe that the individual difference variables of NA, perfectionism, and Type A personality will moderate the leader's workaholism to leader outcomes relationship through systematic increases in and reactions to workaholic perceptions and behaviors resulting in stronger negative well-being consequences. While there is no empirical literature testing these propositions, there is support from the greater personality and individual difference literature. For example, Clark, Lelchook, and Taylor (2010) found that NA shared unique variance with workaholism above and beyond common conceptions of personality and individual differences.

### Followers' Well-Being Outcomes

Leaders' workaholism not only can negatively influence their own well-being, but also their followers' well-being. Given that leaders and followers are part of the same social system (Moos, 1984), they are inherently linked to one another and as a result, changes in one member of the social system will influence the others. As we have illustrated in Fig. 1, leaders' workaholism can influence follower well-being through two distinct pathways, both of which draw on crossover theory (Westman, 2001, 2011). The difference in these two pathways speaks to the content of "what" is being transmitted from leader to follower.

Via one pathway, we suggest that the expression of workaholism itself can be transmitted to followers, impacting their well-being. We define this phenomenon as workaholic crossover. Leveraging the core dimensions of the workaholism construct we defined earlier, we provide several avenues through which affective, cognitive, and behavioral components of workaholism may directly influence the well-being of followers. Via the second pathway, we suggest that the strain resulting from leaders' workaholism influences followers' well-being, following a more traditional strain—strain crossover approach, for which there is a great deal of empirical support (Bakker, Le Blanc, & Schaufeli, 2005; Bakker, Van Emmerik, & Euwema, 2006; Westman & Etzion, 1999). We address each pathway in turn.

*Crossover of Leaders' Workaholism to Followers' Well-being*

Given that workaholism is a readily observable phenomenon in the work-place, it stands to reason that the expression of workaholism by a leader can influence follower well-being in several ways. Several diverse areas of the literature also lend support to this notion. For example, leaders serve an important role in the organization, demonstrating what organizational values and success look like (Lord & Brown, 2001), signaling the amount of attention that followers are likely to pay to patterns of thinking and behavior expressed by leaders. There are also powerful social processes that tend to bring leader and follower behavior more in line with one another, including notions of prototypicality and group convergence (Ellemers, De Gilder, & Haslam, 2004; Lord, Brown, Harvey, & Hall, 2001) and various contagion process that impact members of proximate social environments (Bono & Ilies, 2006; Johnson, 2009). Whether the components of workaholism that a leader exhibits are adopted as the prototypical standard or simply "caught" by followers, there is strong reason to suggest the influence of workaholism on follower well-being. To guide theorizing, we discuss workaholic crossover as it may occur through the three primary components (i.e., affective, cognitive, and behavioral) of workaholism discussed earlier, and how each of these components may influence follower well-being.

*Affective Workaholic Crossover*

The first pathway through which leader workaholism is likely to have an effect on followers' well-being centers around the transfer of affect and emotions from leader to follower. There is a strong body of literature documenting the effects of emotional contagion across individuals in general (Barsade, 2002; Hatfield, Cacioppo, & Rapson, 1994), and specifically between leaders and followers (Johnson, 2009; Rajah, Song, & Arvey, 2011). As stated earlier, the negative emotions of guilt and anxiety are among the dominant emotions involved in workaholism. Moreover, research has linked workaholism to the experience of negative trait and state affect (Clark et al., 2014). Leaders' negative moods and emotions influence not only the moods of followers, but also how they think, feel, and act (George, 2000). For example, Sy, Côté, and Saavedra (2005) studied the effect of leader mood on team mood and group processes, and found that when the leader was in a negative mood, their groups had a more negative affective tone. This emotional contagion also had detrimental effects on group processes, such that groups with leaders in a negative mood exerted more effort and exhibited worse coordination compared to groups with leaders in a positive mood. Johnson (2008) examined the emotional contagion process between principals and teachers, finding that principal NA was related to lower teacher positive affect at work for teachers high in susceptibility to emotional contagion.

## Cognitive Workaholic Crossover

Leader workaholism may also influence follower well-being through cognitive crossover. Crossover from leader to follower can also stem from the cognitive dimension of workaholism, which involves persistent and frequent thoughts about working. This may have a number of effects on the leader–follower relationships. For instance, one may consider instances of both task intrusion and work–life intrusion, where a workaholic leader may interrupt a subordinate's current task to ask about some unrelated task upon which the leader is perseverating; that same intrusion may come after work hours, requiring the subordinate to develop a response and thus cognitively engage in the work. There is some evidence that this may be more likely to occur when the workaholic leader experiences more work–family conflict him or herself, placing additional strain on subordinates (O'Neill et al., 2009).

## Behavioral Workaholic Crossover

A leader's long working hours may have potentially negative impacts on followers' own behaviors with respect to their work. Borrowing from the literature on implicit and explicit norms (e.g., Taggar & Ellis, 2007; Weiss, 1977), one may expect a workaholic leader's behaviors to be reflected in the behaviors of his or her subordinates. For example, at the organizational level, when organizations have a climate for technology assisted supplemental work, employees were more likely to use communication technology for work purposes at night or on weekends (Fenner & Renn, 2010). Research has shown that when employees try and resist managerial expectations, they may face consequences such as lower performance evaluations or less opportunity for advancement (Perlow, 1998). Given this, employees with a

workaholic leader may be more likely to also engage in workaholic behaviors because of implicit and explicit norms and expectations, as well as to
avoid negative consequences of resisting such expectations.

*Crossover of Leaders' Well-Being to Followers' Well-Being*

Earlier in the chapter we described several negative well-being outcomes
likely to be experienced by workaholic leaders, including decreased job and
life satisfaction, increased stress, burnout, and work–life conflict, and
decreased physical and mental health. Drawing from crossover theory
(Westman, 2001, 2011) and the idea that psychological strain can affect the
strain of another person, we propose that the negative work, family, and
individual well-being outcomes discussed earlier will crossover and negatively influence followers' well-being. Although most of the crossover
research has investigated strain crossover between spouses and cohabitat-
ing, there have been some studies investigating crossover within the workplace between leaders and followers. Additionally, given that leaders are
salient role models, crossover effects may be particularly pronounced
between leaders and followers (O'Neill et al., 2009).

The first set of negative leader well-being outcomes discussed in the present chapter includes work-related well-being outcomes (e.g., job satisfaction, job stress, job burnout). Leader–follower crossover of these well-being
outcomes has been demonstrated across several studies. For example,
Westman and Etzion (1999) investigated crossover on a sample of school
principals and teachers, finding that leaders' job-induced tension influenced
teachers' reports of job-induced strain. Although they did not specifically
examine leader job satisfaction, Hinkin, Holtom, and Liu (2012) found that
unit-level job satisfaction change affected an individual unit member's job
satisfaction change over a two year period. Empirical work also supports the
crossover of leader burnout to follower burnout (e.g., Price & Weiss, 2000).
Recently, Ten Brummelhuis, Haar, and Roche (2014) examined a sample of
199 leaders and 456 followers across time, and found that leader burnout
was related to follower burnout, and that this relationship was mediated by
decreased leader supportive behaviors. Additionally, Hakanen, Perhoniemi,
and Bakker (2014) examined 470 Finnish dentist–dental nurse dyads and
found that the dentists' burnout was related to levels of the dental nurses'
burnout, particularly when collaboration was frequent. Interestingly, the
dentists (leaders) were not affected by the dental nurses' (followers) burnout,

suggesting that the hierarchical nature of the leader–follower relationship facilitates top-down rather than bottom-up crossover.

The second set of negative leader well-being outcomes that may cross-over to the follower includes family-related well-being outcomes (e.g., family satisfaction, work–family conflict). Much of the work–family cross-over research has focused on crossover between partners, rather than between leaders and followers, this body of research has shown clear evidence that when one partner experience work–family conflict, this can also increase work–family conflict for their partners (Bakker, Demerouti, & Dollard, 2008; Matthews, Del Priore, Acitelli, & Barnes-Farrell, 2006). While leaders' work–family conflict was not specifically examined, van Emmerik and Peeters (2009) found evidence that team-level work–family conflict and family–work conflict influenced individual-level work–family conflict and family–work conflict, respectively.

The third and final set of negative leader well-being outcomes discussed in the present chapter includes several individual outcomes (e.g., life satisfaction, physical, and mental health). Howe, Levy, and Caplan (2004) investigated crossover processes of depressive symptoms between married couples after a job loss, finding that not only do depressive symptoms of each partner cross over to the other partner, but that these depressive symptoms may also be mutually reinforcing. In a study examining these crossover processes at work, Barnes, Lucianetti, Bhave, and Christian (2015) examined leader–follower crossover using an experience sampling methodology and found poor nightly leader sleep quality was related to lower daily subordinate unit work engagement, and this process was mediated through leader ego depletion and daily abusive supervisor behaviors. Each of these unique crossover pathways may be expected to contribute to negative well-being outcomes for followers of workaholic leaders, especially in light of potential moderating variables discussed in the following section.

### Contextual Moderators

There are a number of potential contextual variables that may ultimately influence the extent to which workaholic crossover and well-being (strain–strain crossover) are experienced. Particularly noteworthy, given the parallel interest in the general workaholic and leadership literatures, is the nature of the work environment and the specific climates or cultures created within that environment. Perhaps one of the more important considerations for the workaholic leader stems from characteristics of the current work environment, characteristics of the broader industry and the nature of responsibility spanning leader and follower roles in getting work accomplished. Furthermore, one must consider the role that task structure and other attributes may have on either mitigating or exacerbating outcomes related to workaholic leaders and their followers. Another critical contextual factor to consider stems from the specific climates that are created at the group level, and the culture of the organization as a whole. Specific cultures for competitiveness or achievement may exacerbate the workaholic leader−follower relationship. Additionally, group climates and norms may also form a contributing role, carrying the expectations of how and when individuals ought to be working (e.g., Fenner & Renn, 2010).

## FUTURE DIRECTIONS

We encourage additional research examining workaholism in relation to leader−follower relationships. Researchers have called for additional attention to the important role leaders play in fostering followers' employee engagement (Shuck & Herd, 2012), and we similarly encourage researchers to examine not only what leadership behaviors influence the well-being of followers, but also what leader behaviors influence the development of follower workaholism. Recent studies have examined the role of leadership in fostering followers' work engagement (De Clercq, Bouckenooghe, Raja, & Matsyborska, 2014). For example, Tims, Bakker, and Xanthopoulou (2011) found that transformational leaders can foster daily work engagement in followers though enhancement of followers' personal resources (e.g., increased follower optimism). To date we are not aware of research studies examining the role of leadership styles or behaviors in fostering workaholism in followers (at either the between- or within-level). These studies could also have important practical implications. For example, organizations may be able to offset the degree to which leaders' workaholic behaviors (e.g., not disengaging from work during non-work hours) foster similar behavioral patterns in their subordinates by setting firm expectations on how often employees are expected to check their work e-mail (e.g., not requiring employees to check work e-mail on weekends). Future research is needed to understand the possible mechanisms (e.g., resource drain; ego depletion) through which different leader behaviors and styles foster employees' workaholism. Additionally, as articulated in our conceptual model, leaders' workaholism may negatively influence not only their own well-being, but the well-being of their followers through various crossover processes;

however, to date there are no studies that have examined these proposed mechanisms.

Related to the above point, not only is additional research needed, we encourage researchers to utilize a variety of methodologies to better understand how these relationships may play out over time (e.g., using longitudinal designs) or on a momentary level (e.g., using an experience sampling methodology). Longitudinal designs could clarify how relationships between workaholism and leadership emerge. For example, are workaholics more likely to advance into a leadership position because of their workaholic tendencies (e.g., staying at work late into the night), or do the expectations and demands of holding a leadership position encourage and reinforce workaholic tendencies? Additionally, if workaholism becomes more detrimental over time (Ng et al., 2007), then we would expect the negative relationships between leader workaholism and leader/follower well-being outcomes to increase over time. This may be particularly likely if the organization or industry fosters a culture of overwork, or if the follower is also a workaholic, and the leader and follower workaholic tendencies are mutually reinforcing (e.g., a negative spiral). Additionally, drawing from prior research showing leaders can influence daily levels of employee work engagement (Tims et al., 2011), it is possible that leaders can also influence daily levels of follower workaholism. Future research should examine this possibility by examining leader–follower relationships at the daily level. This type of methodology allows for the simultaneous examination of leader or organization factors (e.g., the leader's level of workaholism, leader behaviors, organizational culture) and momentary factors (e.g., daily expectations for excessive work, affective, and cognitive processes) to better understand how various factors may influence followers' workaholism as well as implications for their well-being. Another valuable avenue would be to further address workaholic dynamics related to multiple levels of analysis. Such research could provide insight not only into the relationships between a leader and different followers, but also in the interactions between the followers themselves, and how workaholism relates to well-being outcomes at the individual and collective levels of analysis.

While we attempted to provide a comprehensive model outlining the relationship between leader workaholism and well-being outcomes, there are likely many other variables that can be considered. For example, it may also be important to consider followers' perceptions regarding the legitimacy of the workaholism expressed by a leader. Based in the fact that leadership positions often involve more responsibility and greater sacrifice, the extent to which followers perceive a certain degree of workaholism as a necessary or even expected pattern among leaders needs to be considered. Embedded within this perspective is also the degree to which followers perceive their own roles and responsibilities as requiring the same degree of workaholism as accompanying higher levels in the organization. Both of these factors may greatly influence the types and boundary conditions of interactions between leaders and their followers. Also, characteristics of the workers themselves may moderate the leader—follower crossover processes. For example, if a follower is also a workaholic, this may foster a negative feedback loop in which the workaholic tendencies of the leader and follower are mutually reinforcing.

## CONCLUSION

Workaholism is an understudied concept in organizational behavior, and particularly in a leadership context. However, leaders' workaholism can have profound negative effects both on their own well-being as well as the well-being of their followers, as they serve as salient role models for those around them and have the potential to shape followers' healthy (i.e., work engagement) or unhealthy (i.e., workaholism) investment in work. We hope our conceptual model provides a framework that future researchers can utilize to examine these relationships.

## REFERENCES

Andreassen, C. S., Hetland, J., Molde, H., & Pallesen, S. (2011). 'Workaholism' and potential outcomes in well-being and health in a cross-occupational sample. *Stress and Health*, *27*, 209–214.

Andreassen, C. S., Hetland, J., & Pallesen, S. (2010). The relationship between workaholism, basic needs satisfaction at work and personality. *European Journal of Personality*, *24*, 3–17.

Andreassen, C. S., Hetland, J., & Pallesen, S. (2013). Workaholism and work-family spillover in a cross-occupational sample. *European Journal of Work and Organizational Psychology*, *22*, 78–87.

Andreassen, C. S., Ursin, H., Eriksen, H. R., & Pallesen, S. (2012). The relationship of narcissism with workaholism, work engagement, and professional position. *Social Behavior and Personality*, *40*, 881–890.

Avolio, B. J. (2007). Promoting more integrative strategies for leadership theory-building. *American Psychologist*, *62*, 25–33.

Avolio, B. J., Bass, B. M., & Jung, D. I. (1999). Re-examining the components of transformational and transactional leadership using the multifactor leadership questionnaire. *Journal of Occupational and Organizational Psychology*, *72*, 441–462.

Aziz, S., & Zickar, M. J. (2006). A cluster analysis investigation of workaholism as a syndrome. *Journal of Occupational Health Psychology*, *11*, 52–62.

Bakker, A. B., Demerouti, E., & Burke, R. (2009). Workaholism and relationship quality: A spillover-crossover perspective. *Journal of Occupational Health Psychology*, *14*, 23–33.

Bakker, A. B., Demerouti, E., & Dollard, M. F. (2008). How job demands affect partners' experience of exhaustion: Integrating work-family conflict and crossover theory. *Journal of Applied Psychology*, *93*, 901–911.

Bakker, A. B., Le Blanc, P. M., & Schaufeli, W. B. (2005). Burnout contagion among nurses who work at intensive care units. *Journal of Advanced Nursing*, *51*, 276–287.

Bakker, A. B., Van Emmerik, I. J. H., & Euwema, M. C. (2006). Crossover of burnout and engagement in work teams. *Work and Occupations*, *33*, 464–489.

Balducci, C., Cecchin, M., Fraccaroli, F., & Schaufeli, W. B. (2012). Exploring the relationship between workaholism and workplace aggressive behaviour: The role of job-related emotion. *Personality and Individual Differences*, *53*, 629–634.

Barnes, C. M., Lucianetti, L., Bhave, D. P., & Christian, M. S. (2015). You wouldn't like me when I'm sleepy: Leader sleep, daily abusive supervision, and work unit engagement. *Academy of Management Journal*, *58*, 1419–1437.

Barrick, M. R., & Mount, M. K. (2005). Yes, personality matters: Moving on to more important matters. *Human Performance*, *18*, 359–372.

Barsade, S. (2002). The ripple effect: Emotional contagion and its influence on group behavior. *Administrative Science Quarterly*, *47*, 644–675.

Bartczak, M., & Ogińska-Bulik, N. (2012). Workaholism and mental health among Polish academic workers. *International Journal of Occupational Safety and Ergonomics*, *18*, 3–13.

Baruch, Y. (2011). The positive wellbeing aspects of workaholism in cross cultural perspective: The chocoholism metaphor. *Career Development International*, *16*, 572–591.

Bass, B. M. (1999). Two decades of research and development in transformational leadership. *European Journal of Work and Organizational Psychology*, *8*, 9–32.

Bass, B. M., & Avolio, B. J. (1995). *The multifactor leadership questionnaire (MLQ)*. Redwood City, CA: Mind Garden.

Berry, C., Ones, D., & Sackett, P. (2007). Interpersonal deviance, organizational deviance, and their common correlates: A review and meta-analysis. *Journal of Applied Psychology*, *92*, 410–424.

Blair-Loy, M. (2003). *Competing devotions: Career and family among women executives*. Cambridge, MA: Harvard University Press.

Bluen, S. D., Barling, J., & Burns, W. (1990). Predicting sales performance, job satisfaction, and depression by using the achievement strivings and impatience-irritability dimensions of Type A behavior. *Journal of Applied Psychology*, *75*, 212–216.

Bono, J. E., & Ilies, R. (2006). Charisma, positive emotions, and mood contagion. *The Leadership Quarterly*, *17*, 317–334.

Bono, J. E., & Judge, T. A. (2004). Personality and transformational and transactional leadership: A meta-analysis. *Journal of Applied Psychology*, *89*, 901–910.

Brady, B. R., Vodanovich, S. J., & Rotunda, R. (2008). The impact of workaholism of work-family conflict, job satisfaction, & perception of leisure activities. *The Psychologist-Manager Journal*, *11*, 241–263.

Brett, J. M., & Stroh, L. K. (2003). Working 61 plus hours a week: Why do managers do it? *Journal of Applied Psychology, 88*, 67−78.

Burke, R. J. (1999). Workaholism and extra-work satisfactions. *International Journal of Organizational Analysis, 7*, 352−364.

Burke, R. J. (2001). Workaholism components, job satisfaction, and career progress. *Journal of Applied Social Psychology, 31*, 2339−2356.

Burke, R. J., & Fiksenbaum, L. (2009). Work motivations, satisfactions, and health among managers passion versus addiction. *Cross-Cultural Research, 43*, 349−365.

Burke, R. J., Matthiesen, S. B., & Pallesen, S. (2006). Personality correlates of workaholism. *Personality and Individual Differences, 40*, 1223−1233.

Chen, G., Kirkman, B. L., Kanfer, R., Allen, D., & Rosen, B. (2007). A multilevel study of leadership, empowerment, and performance in teams. *Journal of Applied Psychology, 92*, 331−346.

Christian, M. S., Garza, A. S., & Slaughter, J. E. (2011). Work engagement: A quantitative review and test of its relations with task and contextual performance. *Personnel Psychology, 64*, 89−136.

Clark, M. A., Hunter, E. M., Beiler-May, A. A., & Carlson, D. S. (2015, April). An examination of daily workaholism: Causes and consequences. Paper presented at the annual meeting of the Society for Industrial and Organizational Psychology, Philadelphia, PA.

Clark, M. A., Lelchook, A. M., & Taylor, M. L. (2010). Beyond the big five: How narcissism, perfectionism, and dispositional affect relate to workaholism. *Personality and Individual Differences, 48*, 786−791.

Clark, M. A., Michel, J. S., Stevens, G. W., Howell, J. W., & Scruggs, R. S. (2014). Workaholism, work engagement, and work-home outcomes: Exploring the mediating role of positive and negative emotions. *Stress and Health, 30*, 287−300.

Clark, M. A., Michel, J. S., Zhdanova, L., Pui, S., & Baltes, B. B. (2014). All work and no play? A meta-analytic examination of the correlates and outcomes of workaholism. *Journal of Management.* Advance online publication. doi: 10.1177/0149206314522301

Cohan, W. D. (2015, October 3). Deaths draw attention to Wall Street's grueling pace. *New York Times.* Retrieved from http://nyti.ms/1PUQDtL

Deal, J. J. (2015). *Always on, never done? Don't blame the smartphone.* [White Paper]. Greensboro, NC: Center for Creative Leadership. Retrieved from http://insights.ccl.org/wp-content/uploads/2015/04/AlwaysOn.pdf

De Clercq, D., Bouckenooghe, D., Raja, U., & Matsyborska, G. (2014). Servant leadership and work engagement: The contingency effects of leader-follower social capital. *Human Resource Development Quarterly, 25*, 183−212.

De Cremer, D., & Van Dijk, E. (2005). When and why leaders put themselves first: Leader behaviour in resource allocations as a function of feeling entitled. *European Journal of Social Psychology, 35*, 553−563.

Deci, E. L., & Ryan, R. M. (1985). *Intrinsic motivation and self-determination in human behavior.* New York, NY: Plenum.

DeRue, D. S., Nahrgang, J. D., Wellman, N., & Humphrey, S. E. (2011). Trait and behavioral theories of leadership: An integration and meta-analytic test of their relative validity. *Personnel Psychology, 64*, 7−52.

Eagly, A. H. (1987). *Sex differences in social behavior: A social-role interpretation.* Hillsdale, NJ: Erlbaum.

Edwards, J. R., & Baglioni, A. J. (1991). Relationship between type a behavior pattern and mental and physical symptoms: A comparison of global and component measures. *Journal of Applied Psychology, 76,* 276–290.

Edwards, J. R., & Rothbard, N. P. (2000). Mechanisms linking work and family: Clarifying the relationship between work and family constructs. *The Academy of Management Review, 25,* 178–199.

Elfenbein, H. A. (2007). Emotion in organizations: A review and theoretical integration. *Academy of Management Annals, 1,* 315–386.

Ellemers, N., De Gilder, D., & Haslam, S. A. (2004). Motivation individuals and groups at work a social identity perspective on leadership and group performance. *Academy of Management Review, 29,* 459–478.

Ezzedeen, S. R., & Swiercz, P. M. (2007). Development and initial validation of a cognitive-based work-nonwork conflict scale. *Psychological Reports, 100,* 979–999.

Fassel, D. (1990). *Working ourselves to death: The high costs of workaholism, the rewards of recovery.* San Francisco, CA: Harper Collins.

Fenner, G. H., & Renn, R. W. (2010). Technology-assisted supplemental work and work-to-family conflict: The role of instrumentality beliefs, organizational expectations and time management. *Human Relations, 63,* 63–82.

Gallup. (2014). *The "40-hour" workweek is actually longer.* Retrieved from http://www.gallup.com/poll/175286/hour-workweek-actually-longer-seven-hours.aspx

George, J. M. (2000). Emotions and leadership: The role of emotional intelligence. *Human Relations, 53,* 1027–1055.

Graves, L. M., Ruderman, M. N., Ohlott, P. J., & Weber, T. J. (2012). Driven to work and enjoyment of work: Effects on managers' outcomes. *Journal of Management, 38,* 1655–1680.

Greenhaus, J. H., & Beutell, N. J. (1985). Sources of conflict between work and family roles. *Academy of Management Review, 10,* 76–88.

Greenhause, S. (2001, September 1). Report shows Americans have more 'Labor Days'. *New York Times,* p. A6.

Hakanen, J. J., Perhoniemi, R., & Bakker, A. B. (2014). Crossover of exhaustion between dentists and dental nurses. *Stress and Health, 30,* 110–121.

Harris, K. J., Marett, K., & Harris, R. B. (2011). Technology-related pressure and work-family conflict: Main effects and an examination of moderating variables. *Journal of Applied Social Psychology, 41,* 2077–2103.

Hatfield, E., Cacioppo, J. T., & Rapson, R. L. (1994). *Emotional contagion: Studies in emotion and social interaction.* Cambridge, UK: Cambridge University Press.

Hinkin, T. R., Holtom, B., & Liu, D. (2012). The contagion effect: Understanding the impact of changes in individual and work-unit satisfaction on hospitality industry turnover. *Cornell Hospitality Reports, 12,* 6–12.

Hogan, R. (1991). Personality and personality measurement. In M. D. Dunnette & L. M. Hough (Eds.), *The handbook of industrial and organizational psychology* (2nd ed., Vol. 2, pp. 873–919). Palo Alto, CA: Consulting Psychologists Press.

Hogan, R. (2005). In defense of personality measurement: New wine for old whiners. *Human Performance, 18,* 331–341.

Howe, G. W., Levy, M. L., & Caplan, R. D. (2004). Job loss and depressive symptoms in couples: Common stressors, stress transmission, or relationship disruption? *Journal of Family Psychology, 18,* 639–650.

Huang, X., Iun, J., Liu, A., & Gong, Y. (2010). Does participative leadership enhance work performance by inducing empowerment or trust? The differential effects on managerial and non-managerial subordinates. *Journal of Organizational Behavior, 31*, 122−143.

Johnson, S. K. (2008). I second that emotion: Effects of emotional contagion and affect at work on leader and follower outcomes. *The Leadership Quarterly, 19*, 1−19.

Johnson, S. K. (2009). Do you feel what I feel? Mood contagion and leadership outcomes. *The Leadership Quarterly, 20*, 814−827.

Judge, T. A., Piccolo, R. F., & Ilies, R. (2004). The forgotten ones? The validity of consideration and initiating structure in leadership research. *Journal of Applied Psychology, 89*, 36−51.

Kahn, R. L., & Byosiere, P. (1992). Stress in organizations. In M. D. Dunnette & L. M. Hough (Eds.), *Handbook of industrial and organizational psychology* (2nd ed., Vol. 3, pp. 571−650). Palo Alto, CA: Consulting Psychologists Press.

Kuhn, P., & Lozano, F. (2008). The expanding workweek? Understanding trends in long work hours among U.S. men, 1979−2006. *Journal of Labor Economics, 26*, 311−343.

Lavine, L. (2014, November 18). Why you should stop bragging about being a workaholic. *Fast Company*. Retrieved from http://www.fastcompany.com/3038640/why-should-stop-bragging-about-being-a-workaholic

Lord, R. G., & Brown, D. J. (2001). Leadership, values, and subordinate self-concepts. *The Leadership Quarterly, 12*, 133−152.

Lord, R. G., Brown, D. J., Harvey, J. L., & Hall, R. J. (2001). Contextual constraints on prototype generation and their multilevel consequences for leadership perceptions. *The Leadership Quarterly, 12*, 311−338.

Machlowitz, M. M. (1978). *Determining the effects of workaholism*. Doctoral dissertation. Available from ProQuest Dissertations and Theses database. UMI No. 7915855.

Maslach, C., Schaufeli, W. B., & Leiter, M. P. (2001). Job burnout. *Annual Review of Psychology, 52*, 397−422.

Matthews, R. A., Del Priore, R. E., Acitelli, L. K., & Barnes-Farrell, J. L. (2006). Work-to relationship conflict: Crossover effects in dual-earner couples. *Journal of Occupational Health Psychology, 11*, 228−240.

McCauley, C. D. (2004). Successful and unsuccessful leadership. In J. Antonakis, A. T. Cianciolo, & R. J. Sternberg (Eds.), *The nature of leadership* (pp. 199−221). Thousand Oaks, CA: Sage Publications.

Meinert, D. (2014, August). 5 types of bad bosses: Can they be fixed? *HR Magazine, 59*, 26−32.

Moos, R. (1984). Context and coping: Toward a unifying conceptual framework. *American Journal of Community Psychology, 12*, 5−25.

Murphy, L. R., & Sauter, S. L. (2003). The USA perspective: Current issues and trends in the management of work stress. *Australian Psychologist, 38*, 151−157.

Ng, T. W. H., Sorensen, K. L., & Feldman, D. C. (2007). Dimensions, antecedents, and consequences of workaholism: A conceptual integration and extension. *Journal of Organizational Behavior, 28*, 111−136.

Oates, W. E. (1971). *Confessions of a workaholic: The facts about work addiction*. New York, NY: World.

O'Neill, J. W., Harrison, M. M., Cleveland, J., Almeida, D., Stawski, R., & Crouter, A. C. (2009). Work−family climate, organizational commitment, and turnover: Multilevel contagion effects of leaders. *Journal of Vocational Behavior, 74*, 18−29.

Organization and Economic Cooperation and Development. (2015). *OECD.* Stat (LFS – Average Annual Hours Worked). Accessed on October 18, 2015.

Peiperl, M., & Jones, B. (2001). Workaholics and overworkers: Productivity or pathology? *Group and Organization Management, 26*, 369–393.

Perlow, L. A. (1998). Boundary control: The social ordering of work and family time in a high-tech corporation. *Administrative Science Quarterly, 43*, 328–357.

Porter, G. (2006). Profiles of workaholism among high-tech managers. *Career Development International, 11*, 440–462.

Price, M. S., & Weiss, M. R. (2000). Relationships among coach burnout, coach behaviours, and athletes' psychological responses. *Sport Psychologist, 14*, 391–409.

Rajah, R., Song, Z., & Arvey, R. D. (2011). Emotionality and leadership: Taking stock of the past decade of research. *The Leadership Quarterly, 22*, 1107–1119.

Robinson, B. E. (1998). *Chained to the desk: A guidebook for workaholics, their partners and children and the clinicians who treat them.* New York, NY: New York University Press.

Robinson, B. E. (2000). A typology of workaholics with implications for counselors. *Journal of Addictions & Offender Counseling, 21*, 34–48.

Robinson, B. E., & Post, P. (1995). Work addiction as a function of family of origin and its influence on current family functioning. *The Family Journal: Counseling and Therapy for Couples and Families, 3*, 200–206.

Schaufeli, W. B., Bakker, A. B., van der Heijden, F. M. M. A., & Prins, J. T. (2009a). Workaholism among medical residents: It the combination of working excessively and compulsively that counts. *International Journal of Stress Management, 16*, 249–272.

Schaufeli, W. B., Bakker, A. B., van der Heijden, F. M. M. A., & Prins, J. T. (2009b). Workaholism, burnout, and well-being among junior doctors: The mediating role of role conflict. *Work and Stress, 23*, 155–172.

Schaufeli, W. B., Salanova, M., González-Romá, V., & Bakker, A. B. (2002). The measurement of engagement and burnout: A confirmative analytic approach. *Journal of Happiness Studies, 3*, 71–92.

Schaufeli, W. B., Taris, T. W., & Bakker, A. B. (2008). It takes two to tango: Workaholism is working excessively and working compulsively. In R. J. Burke & C. L. Cooper (Eds.), *The long work hours culture: Causes, consequences and choices* (pp. 203–225). Bingley, UK: Emerald Group Publishing Limited.

Schaufeli, W. B., Taris, T. W., & Van Rhenen, W. (2008). Workaholism, burnout, and work engagement: Three of a kind or three different kinds of employee well-being? *Applied Psychology: An International Review, 57*, 173–203.

Schor, J. (2003). The (even more) overworked American. In de Graaf (Ed.), *Take back your time: Fighting overwork and time poverty in America* (pp. 6–11). San Francisco, CA: Berrett-Koehler Publishers, Inc.

Scott, K. S., Moore, K. S., & Miceli, M. P. (1997). An exploration of the meaning and consequences of workaholism. *Human Relations, 50*, 287–314.

Shuck, B., & Herd, A. M. (2012). Employee engagement and leadership: Exploring the convergence of two frameworks and implications for leadership development in HRD. *Human Resource Development Review, 11*, 156–181.

Singal, J. (2014, November 4). Workaholism is really bad for you. *Yahoo Health.* Retrieved from https://www.yahoo.com/health/workaholism-is-really-bad-for-you-101759990467.html

Slaney, R. B., Rice, K. G., Mobley, M., Trippi, J., & Ashby, J. S. (2001). The revised almost perfect scale. *Measurement and Evaluation in Counseling and Development, 34*, 130–145.

Smith, D. E., & Seymour, R. B. (2004). The nature of addiction. In R. H. Coombs (Ed.), *Handbook of addictive disorders: A practical guide to diagnosis and treatment* (pp. 3–30). Hoboken, NJ: John Wiley & Sons, Inc.

Snir, R., & Harpaz, I. (2012). Beyond workaholism: Towards a general model of heavy work investment. *Human Resource Management Review, 22*, 232–243.

Somech, A. (2003). Relationships of participative leadership with relational demography variables: A multi-level perspective. *Journal of Organizational Behavior, 24*, 1003–1018.

Sonnentag, S., Mojza, E. J., Binnewies, C., & Scholl, A. (2008). Being engaged at work and detached at home: A week-level study on work engagement, psychological detachment, and affect. *Work & Stress, 22*, 257–276.

Spector, P. E. (1997). *Job satisfaction: Applications, assessment, causes and consequences.* Thousand Oaks, CA: Sage.

Spence, J. T., & Robbins, A. S. (1992). Workaholism: Definition, measurement, and preliminary results. *Journal of Personality Assessment, 58*, 160–178.

Stillman, J. (2014, November 11). *Why you shouldn't be proud to be a workaholic.* Inc. Retrieved from http://www.inc.com/jessica-stillman/why-you-shouldn-t-be-proud-to-be-a-workaholic.html

Sy, T., Côté, S., & Saavedra, R. (2005). The contagious leader: Impact of the leader's mood on the mood of group members, group affective tone, and group processes. *Journal of Applied Psychology, 90*, 295–305.

Taggar, S., & Ellis, R. (2007). The role of leaders in shaping formal team norms. *The Leadership Quarterly, 18*, 105–120.

Taris, T. W., Geurts, S. A. E., Schaufeli, W. B., Blonk, R. W. B., & Lagerveld, S. E. (2008). All day and all of the night: The relative contribution of two dimensions of workaholism to well-being in self-employed workers. *Work & Stress, 22*, 153–165.

Ten Brummelhuis, L. L., Haar, J. M., & Roche, M. (2014). Does family life help to be a better leader? A closer look at crossover processes from leaders to followers. *Personnel Psychology, 67*, 917–949.

Tims, M., Bakker, A. B., & Xanthopoulou, D. (2011). Do transformational leaders enhance their followers' daily work engagement? *The Leadership Quarterly, 22*, 121–131.

van Beek, I., Hu, Q., Schaufeli, Q. B., Taris, T. W., & Schreurs, B. H. J. (2012). For fun, love, or money: What drives workaholic, engaged, and burned-out employees at work? *Applied Psychology: An International Review, 61*, 30–55.

van Beek, I., Taris, T. W., & Schaufeli, W. B. (2011). Workaholic and work engaged employees: Dead ringers or worlds apart? *Journal of Occupational Health Psychology, 16*, 468–482.

van Beek, I., Taris, T. W., Schaufeli, W. B., & Brenninkmeijer, V. (2014). Heavy work investment: Its motivational make-up and outcomes. *Journal of Managerial Psychology, 49*, 46–62.

van Emmerik, I. J. H., & Peeters, M. C. W. (2009). Crossover specificity of team-level work-family conflict to individual-level work-family conflict. *Journal of Managerial Psychology, 24*, 254–268.

Van Wijhe, C. I., Peeters, M. C. W., & Schaufeli, W. B. (2014). Enough is enough: Cognitive antecedents of workaholism and its aftermath. *Human Resource Management, 53*, 157–177.

Watson, D., & Clark, L. A. (1992). Affects separable and inseparable: On the hierarchical arrangement of the negative affects. *Journal of Personality and Social Psychology*, *62*, 489–505.

Weiss, H. M. (1977). Subordinate imitation of supervisor behavior: The role of modeling in organizational socialization. *Organizational Behavior and Human Performance*, *19*, 89–105.

Westman, M. (2001). Stress and strain crossover. *Human Relations*, *54*, 717–751.

Westman, M. (2011). The impact of stress on the individual, the dyad and the team. *Stress and Health*, *27*, 177–180.

Westman, M., & Etzion, D. (1999). The crossover of strain from school principles to teachers and vice versa. *Journal of Occupational Health Psychology*, *4*, 269–278.

# STRESS, WELL-BEING, AND THE DARK SIDE OF LEADERSHIP

Seth M. Spain, P. D. Harms and Dustin Wood

## ABSTRACT

*The role of dark side personality characteristics in the workplace has received increasing attention in the organizational sciences and from leadership researchers in particular. We provide a review of this area, mapping out the key frameworks for assessing the dark side. We pay particular attention to the roles that the dark side plays in leadership processes and career dynamics, with special attention given to destructive leadership. Further, we examine the role that stress plays in the emergence of leaders and how the dark side plays into that process. We additionally provide discussion of the possible roles that leaders can play in producing stress experiences for their followers. We finally illustrate a dynamic model of the interplay of dark leadership, social relationships, and stress in managerial derailment. Throughout, we emphasize a functionalist account of these personality characteristics, placing particular focus on the motives and emotional capabilities of the individuals under discussion.*

**Keywords:** Dark personality; dark triad; subclinical; leadership; laissez-faire leadership; stress

The Role of Leadership in Occupational Stress
Research in Occupational Stress and Well Being, Volume 14, 33–59
Copyright © 2016 by Emerald Group Publishing Limited
All rights of reproduction in any form reserved
ISSN: 1479-3555/doi:10.1108/S1479-355520160000014002

There is a burgeoning literature in the organizational sciences surrounding what have been called subclinical or "dark" personality characteristics (Hogan & Hogan, 2001; Paulhus & Williams, 2002). These are character traits such as narcissism, psychopathy, or paranoia that cannot be adequately represented as combinations of the "normal" personality traits (e.g., extraversion, agreeableness) found in the Five Factor Model (Digman, 1990; Goldberg, 1993; McCrae & Costa, 1995; Wiggins, 1996) and that are associated with dysfunctional behavioral patterns. This literature has consistently asserted that a relationship exists between stress and so-called "dark side" characteristics. Specifically, it has been argued that the behaviors and tactics typical of individuals high on these dark side traits are not necessarily maladaptive, and may even have positive effects under some conditions. However, their negative attributes become enhanced and tip toward the destructive side of human behavior under conditions of stress. In workplace situations, these responses to stress may trigger a vicious downward spiral as individuals with elevated dark personality traits begin to induce stress in others and possibly provoke hostile responses that only exacerbate the problem. Here, we will discuss the nature of dark side characteristics, detail how stress and uncertainty may provoke destructive patterns of behavior, and how these behaviors may impact the stress and well-being of others.

Our goal is to move beyond purely structuralist interpretations of these personality characteristics and instead take a functionalist approach to understanding dark personality. Functionalist approaches generally emphasize that levels of behavioral and psychological tendencies are shaped by their real or perceived utility to the actor for attaining valued outcomes (Wood, Gardner, & Harms, 2015; cf., Ajzen, 1991; Gintis, 2007). Here, we will focus on how emotional reactance, emotional regulation, and the ability to perceive emotion can be understood as potential antecedents of "dark" characteristics by shaping the perceived functionality of such characteristics to the actor. Specifically, we discuss a functional model of personality that stresses individual's motives, perceptual biases, and emotional (in)capacities as underlying the behavioral regularities assessed by dark personality batteries. Further, we will move beyond decontextualized models of personality to suggest that both the organizational context and coworkers play an important role in the dynamic interplay between dark side personality and stress. Fig. 1 presents our overarching model, which features the sorts of functional antecedents we expect to underlie dark personality characteristics, and shows that dark traits interact with environmental stressors to produce destructive/dysfunctional leader behavior, which in turn, negatively impacts employee well-being.

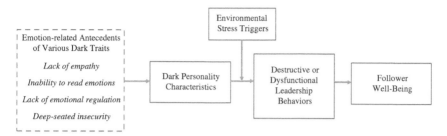

*Fig. 1.* A General Model of Emotions, Stress, and Well-Being for Dark Leadership. *Notes:* We would argue that "dark personality" characteristics are isomorphic to behavioral tendencies that are driven by the emotion-related antecedents. These behavioral tendencies are frequently functional under normal conditions, but stress triggers in the person's environment change the functional value of these behaviors, such that these typical behaviors become dysfunctional at best or destructive at worst. In either case, the expected impact on follower well-being is negative.

## THE DARK SIDE OF PERSONALITY

Most research into dark personality has been conducted in a tradition we call "structuralist," in that it is built on a foundation of factor analytic (structural) personality traits. Much of this research has focused on the three characteristics referred to as the Dark Triad — Machiavellianism, Narcissism, and Psychopathy (Paulhus & Williams, 2002) — though more recent theoretical consideration has expanded this to the "Dark Tetrad" by adding a fourth characteristic, Sadism, to the mix (see Paulhus, 2014, discussed in section "Dark Tetrad"); we will use this more recent framework. The Dark Tetrad approach associated with Paulhus' work is focused on characteristic motives to elevate the self and harm others (Paulhus & Williams, 2002). An alternative approach to dark personality is based on models of DSM-IV Axis II personality disorders (Hogan & Hogan, 2001, 2009), and focuses on the dark side as potentially aversive personality characteristics that emerge when individuals let down their guard (Hogan & Hogan, 2001).

### Dark Tetrad

*Machiavellianism*, which refers to a manipulative personality, based on questioning individuals about how much they agree with statements derived from sentiments and prescriptions for leader behavior in the writings of Niccolo Machiavelli (Christie & Geis, 1970). Machiavellians show a lack of empathy, display little emotion, and hold an unconventional moral perspective. Specifically, they are willing to lie to, manipulate, and exploit other people, and they focus exclusively on their own goals, displaying no concerns about the wishes of others (Christie & Geis, 1970; Wu & LeBreton, 2011). An important distinction is that Machiavellians are exceedingly *willing* to manipulate others, but they are not necessarily *better* at manipulation than non-Machiavellians (Jones & Paulhus, 2009). A defining characteristic of Machiavellians is that they take a certain joy in successfully deceiving others. Their highly cynical worldview tends to be that most other people are stupid and gullible, but at the same time secretly deceitful themselves. Consequently, tricking others into believing lies allows the Machiavellian to affirm their own sense of superiority.

Of the dark side characteristics, *narcissism* has received the most research attention in the organizational sciences (see Campbell, Hoffman, Campbell, & Marchiso, 2011 or Grijalva & Harms, 2014 for an overview). This dimension of dark personality emerged from Raskin and Hall's (1979) attempts to develop a subclinical version of Narcissistic personality disorder. Subclinical narcissism therefore has the same facets as the clinical variant: grandiosity, entitlement, dominance, and superiority. Narcissists are prone to *self-enhancement*; they attempt to present a highly idealized version of themselves (Raskin, Novacek, & Hogan, 1991). This self-enhancement allows them to often appear charming or pleasant in the short term. In the long term, however, narcissists "poison the well"; they have difficulty maintaining successful interpersonal relationships, since they lack trust for others, and are more likely to actively feel and show disdain for others (Morf & Rhodewalt, 2001). This prideful element is key to understanding the *emotional core* of narcissism, in that narcissists feel superior to others, in a way that demands respect and awe from others and may even require them to actively put others down (cf. Horowitz et al., 2006). That said, it has also been argued that there is a second type of narcissist, the vulnerable narcissist, who secretly doubts their own superiority and reacts highly emotionally when challenged (as opposed to grandiose narcissists who tend to ignore negative feedback; see Deluga, 1997; Miller, Gentile, Wilson, & Campbell, 2013).

*Psychopathy* has been described as impulsivity and thrill-seeking combined with low empathy and anxiety (Babiak & Hare, 2006; Hare, 1985; Skeem, Polaschek, Patrick, & Lilienfeld, 2011). *Psychopaths* are characterized as antagonistic and impulsive with a tendency to seek immediate gratification (Cleckley, 1976; Hare, 1999). Further, a major marker of psychopathy is their severely stunted ability to experience and understand emotions, and in particular guilt, anxiety, and empathy (Hare, 1999). Although they may be able to fake displays of appropriate emotions, the feeling underlying that display is essentially alien to them. While psychopathy is characterized by impulsivity at a behavioral level, its core is believed to be the shallowness of affective experience — the classical psychopath as described by Cleckley, Hare, and others, has almost no emotional life, except for brief, intense bursts of anger.

Machiavellianism, narcissism, and psychopathy together comprise what has been called the Dark Triad of personality (Paulhus & Williams, 2002). Paulhus recently suggested the inclusion of *everyday sadism* to the above characteristics (the Dark Tetrad; Buckels, Jones, & Paulhus, 2013; Paulhus, 2014). Sadism is defined most directly by the desire and intention to hurt others, either verbally or physically, simply for the enjoyment of the act. These people cause harm *because they like it*. Sadists simply enjoy seeing others in distress. Paulhus (2014) uses the workplace bully as an example of a classic sadist. As with the other dark characteristics, intimidation and bullying may provide some short-term advantages when competing with others, but ultimately these behaviors undermine social cohesion and reduce the likelihood of forming social bonds in the long term.

Further, Paulhus (2014) provides a discussion of the key features of each of the Dark Tetrad characteristics. As they are typically operationalized, each of the four characteristics includes a mix of negative attributes, but is typically defined by a particular dimension. For example, impulsivity can be considered the cardinal feature of psychopathy, cynicism and concomitant manipulation for Machiavellianism, grandiosity for narcissism, and enjoyment of cruelty for sadism. The common element across *all four* Dark Tetrad characteristics appears to be *callousness* — individuals high on any (set of) Dark Tetrad characteristics tend to lack empathy. They simply do not care about the well-being of other individuals, in general. Paulhus (2014, p. 424) describes the Dark Tetrad as a "callous constellation" to demarcate it from other undesirable personality characteristics. Dark Tetrad characteristics are distinct from one another, and the cardinal feature of each characteristic may point to major pathways different individuals travel to arrive at a lack of concern for others (e.g., mistrust for Machiavellians, and a sense of superiority for Narcissists).

However, the four dimensions also clearly covary; high elevation on one is often accompanied by high elevation on others (Paulhus, 2014). Because of this, a concern with the Dark Tetrad, is whether narcissism,

Machiavellianism, psychopathy, and sadism, are distinct but overlapping constructs or whether they represent alternative manifestation of a deeper latent construct (Jonason & Webster, 2010; Paulhus & Williams, 2002). For instance, as noted above all of the characteristics share an element of callousness (Paulhus, 2014), which may facilitate or underlie all four dimensions.

## Axis II Approaches to Dark Personality

More recent research has focused on subclinical versions of the DSM-IV Axis-II personality disorders (American Psychological Association, 1994), which are often measured with the Hogan Development Survey (HDS; Hogan & Hogan, 2009; cf., Harms, Spain, & Hannah, 2011a; Spain, Harms, & LeBreton, 2014). The HDS assesses what it refers to as 11 personality derailers, which are argued to lead to potential *short-term* advantages, but can cause *long-term* problems (Hogan, 2007; Hogan & Hogan, 2001; Hogan & Kaiser, 2005). These characteristics and their clinical counterparts are listed in Table 1, which also locates the Dark Tetrad characteristics within these frameworks. We aligned Machiavellianism with Paranoid/Skeptical, the best place we could determine for it on the basis of its association with cynicism and distrust. Further, it is unclear to us whether sadism has an alignment within these frameworks − it shares some features with antisocial personality, but that characteristic focuses on the emotional deficit and impulsivity we see as the core of psychopathy. Table 1 also highlights areas we believe most strongly impact individual's in terms of development and stress.

In part because of the desire to use assessments of these dimensions as developmental tools, the HDS uses euphemistic names for its dimensions, in contrast to the rather negatively termed DSM-IV Axis II disorders. It is also worth noting that the HDS uses a dimensional structure as opposed to the categorical diagnoses of the DSM-IV (see also Guenole, 2014 for a discussion of the recently introduced DSM-5). Consider the Skeptical dimension of the HDS. High-scoring Skeptical individuals are viewed as having chips on their shoulders, are cynical, distrustful, easy to anger, and suspicious of others' motives. Individuals scoring low on the Skeptical dimension are perfectly capable of trusting others. High-Skeptical individuals display behavior patterns that are similar to Paranoids, but their behavior is not at so debilitating a level as to necessitate clinical intervention (for a more detailed description of the clinical vs. subclinical distinction the

*Table 1.*　Dark Personality Characteristics and Their Descriptions.

| HDS | DSM-IV | Dark Tetrad | Description of High Scorers (HDS) | DSM-IV Descriptions |
|---|---|---|---|---|
| Excitable | Borderline | | Moody and inconsistent concerns; *being enthusiastic about persons, ideas, and projects and then becoming disappointed in them* | **Inappropriate anger; unstable and intense relationships** |
| Skeptical | Paranoid | Machiavellianism | Cynical, distrustful, *overly sensitive to criticism, and skeptical of others' true intentions* | Distrustful and suspicious of others; motives of others are interpreted negatively |
| Cautious | Avoidant | | *Resistant to change* and reluctant to take even reasonable chances for fear of being evaluated negatively | Social inhibition; feelings of inadequacy; **hypersensitivity to criticism** |
| Reserved | Schizoid | | Socially withdrawn and lacking interest in or awareness of the feelings of others | Emotional coldness and detachment from relationships; indifferent to criticism |
| Leisurely | Passive-Aggressive | | Autonomous, *indifferent to the requests of others,* and often irritable when others persist | **Passive resistance to performance expectations**; irritable when asked to do unwanted tasks |
| Bold | Narcissistic | Narcissism | Unusually self-confident, *unwilling to admit mistakes or listen to advice, and unable to learn from experience* | Grandiose sense of self-importance and entitlement; **arrogant behaviors and attitudes** |
| Mischievous | Antisocial | Psychopathy | **Enjoys taking risks** and testing the limits | **Disregard for the truth; impulsive;** failure to conform to social norms |
| Colorful | Histrionic | | Expressive, dramatic, and desires to be noticed | **Excessive emotionality and attention-seeking** |
| Imaginative | Schizotypal | | Acts and thinks in creative and unusual ways | Odd beliefs and thinking; behavior or speech that is eccentric or peculiar |

*Table 1.* (*Continued*)

| HDS | DSM-IV | Dark Tetrad | Description of High Scorers (HDS) | DSM-IV Descriptions |
|---|---|---|---|---|
| Diligent | Obsessive-Compulsive | | Careful, precise, and critical of the performance of others | Preoccupations with orderliness, rules, and control; **inflexible** |
| Dutiful | Dependent | | Eager to please, *reliant on others for support, and reluctant to take independent action* | **Difficulty making everyday decisions without excessive advice and reassurance;** unwilling to express disagreement |

*Notes*: Machiavellianism is associated with Skeptical/Paranoid due to the core element of distrust of others. We are unable to orient Sadism within this table, since no other characteristic aligns perfectly with its key feature of *enjoyment of cruelty* (Paulhus, 2014). We have italicized elements of characteristics that make them particularly resistant to developmental efforts. Further, we have set elements of characteristics that are likely to be particularly stress-provoking in others in boldface.

reader is directed to LeBreton, Binning, & Adorno, 2006; Wu & LeBreton, 2011).

Subclinical characteristics may pose problems for people high on them under some circumstances (Spain et al., 2014; Wu & LeBreton, 2011), which may include stressful situations, but they do not always hinder day-to-day functioning (Hogan & Hogan, 2001). Under very specific circumstances, these traits may even prove beneficial (e.g., Harms et al., 2011a). These traits have been found to have important consequences for performance (Benson & Campbell, 2007; Harms, Spain, Hannah, Hogan, & Foster, 2011b; O'Boyle, Forsyth, Banks, & McDaniel, 2012), and leader development (Harms et al., 2011a). In spite of these potential advantages, individuals scoring high on these traits are significantly more likely to have trouble with their supervisors, so their behavior is likely a source of concern.

### Honesty—Humility

The last approach we will touch on is the Honesty—humility dimension of the HEXACO model of personality (Ashton et al., 2004). The HEXACO model of personality adds the Honesty—humility dimension to the more common five factors. Honesty—humility can be seen as fairly general lack-of-dark personality, in that it has significant negative correlations with each of the original Dark Triad characteristics (Lee & Ashton, 2005). A high score on Honesty—humility therefore should reflect a probability of relatively low Dark Triad standings. Conversely, a low score on Honesty—humility implies some relatively high Dark Triad standing, though not necessarily on any particular aspect of the Dark Triad, however. This final distinction is important because, as illustrated above, the Dark Triad (and Dark Tetrad, more generally) only completely share one feature: callousness. Hence, low standing on Honesty—humility is likely to imply that they individual is fairly callous, but it does not necessarily provide strong indications about the particular form that this callousness might take. This is one reason we prefer reasonably fine-grained assessments of dark personality, in that more general measures like Honesty—humility are less diagnostic of specific problems.

### Beyond Structuralist Approaches

First, we consider personality characteristics, especially those defined mostly by their behavioral regularities, as in the HDS and HEXACO models, as essentially the same as *behavioral syndromes*: complexes of behaviors that tend to covary across people (cf., Roberts, 2005). Personality characteristics are often conceptually somewhat deeper than this, since they include additional affective and cognitive components. Nonetheless, assessment is typically behavioral, and ultimately it is the actor's behavior which carries the harmful effects of dark psychological characteristics to others. We believe that it is important to expose the underlying *beliefs, motives, abilities*, and *perceptual biases* that drive these behaviors in order to effectively understand and intervene in organizations (e.g., Harms, Spain, & Wood, 2014; see Table 2 for a conceptual sketch of such a model for the Dark Tetrad characteristics). For instance, if a supervisor in our organization is simply classified as narcissistic, we may have considerable difficulty in alleviating the stress that this supervisor is causing his or her subordinates. However, if we understand that the supervisor is motivated to prove his or her excellence by compelling the team to a very high production standard, this should suggest more targeted interventions – for instance, the supervisor may be persuaded to better incentivize employee satisfaction and ease back on the team through an understanding that this will facilitate their more ultimate goal of demonstrating their excellence through the group's achievements.

This approach allows us more "levers" to pull in order to shape the behavior of organizational members. Understanding what motives drive

***Table 2.*** Proposed Motive, Ability, and Perceptual Bias Model for the Dark Tetrad.

| Underlying Mechanism | Narcissism | Machiavellianism | Psychopathy | Sadism |
|---|---|---|---|---|
| Need for Power (Motive) | + + | | + | |
| Need for Affiliation (Motive) | − | − | | − |
| Enjoyment of others suffering (Motive) | | | | + + |
| Capacity to feel empathy (Ability) | − | − | − − | − − |
| Controlling Impulses (Ability) | − | | − − | |
| Positive Perceptions of Others (Perceptual Bias) | − | − − | − | − |
| Positive Views of Self (Perceptual Bias) | + | − | | |

*Notes*: Adapted from Harms et al. (2014). "+" indicates a positive influence of the mechanism on the Dark Tetrad characteristic. "−" indicates a negative influence. No symbol indicates no clear causal connection between the mechanism and the characteristic. Double symbols indicate our belief that the mechanism is a key factor in the characteristic.

employees, what beliefs and perceptual biases color their worldviews, what abilities they have or lack gives the psychologist, human resource manager, or senior leader a more comprehensive understanding of the nature of the problem and the potential avenues for shifting behavior. In contrast, approaching a person as simply "a narcissist" or "a psychopath" provides a label, but is not suggestive of developmental paths. One can design selection systems to try to avoid hiring such people. One can put a psychopath in an "enforcer" role, where they will experience no emotional distress from firing workers (the TV character Jack Donaghy from *30 Rock* certainly never lost any sleep over firing an employee). One could perhaps pair the narcissist with a mentor that the narcissist actually respects, or with a powerful partner who can reign in their behavior, but these selection and organizational structure tools take the standing on the behavioral dimension as a given. If we understand the causes, we can work directly on those causes, changing the behavior, instead of accepting it (Harms, Wood, & Spain, 2016; Harms et al., 2014).

## DARK PERSONALITY AND LEADERSHIP

One of the best established approaches to understanding leadership behaviors is the trait approach to leadership (Hiller, DeChurch, Murase, & Doty, 2011; Zaccaro, 2012). Although the vast majority of this research has been conducted under the paradigm of the Big Five personality traits (Antonakis, Day, & Schyns, 2012) there has been increasing recent calls for more research focusing on dark personality in order to better understand leadership and leader derailment (Harms & Spain, 2015; Hogan & Hogan, 2001; Judge, Piccolo, & Kosalka, 2009; Spain et al., 2014).

The relationship between dark personality characteristics and leadership is more complex than dark personality simply derailing individuals off of their career paths. For example, a number of researchers have suggested that narcissistic tendencies play an important role in both leader successes and failures (e.g., Grijalva, Harms, Newman, Gaddis, & Fraley, 2015; Kets de Vries & Miller, 1985; Rosenthal & Pittinsky, 2006). Beyond this, there is an argument, drawing on evolutionary psychology (e.g., Jonason, Koenig, & Tost, 2010), which suggests that extreme risk-taking behavior, such as that implicated in psychopathy, is often reinforced in organizational leaders because it can lead to success some of the time or in the short term (Johnson, Wrangham, & Rosen, 2002; Jonason et al., 2010). This is in spite of the obvious potential downsides of risk-taking. Naturally, the media have called out such risk-taking since the economic collapse of 2007/2008. That said, studies linking dark personality to leadership outcomes have suggested there is no one-size-fits-all approach – context matters for when dark personality traits play a positive or negative role in leadership (Harms & Spain, 2015; Padilla, Hogan, & Kaiser, 2007).

Studies employing historiometric methods have also shown a positive link between dark personality and leader effectiveness. For example, Machiavellians are effective at forming political alliances and cultivating a charismatic image: a study of 39 US presidents showed that ratings of Machiavellianism were positively associated with not only charisma, but also rated performance (Deluga, 2001). Machiavellian leaders also tend to serve more years in elected office and have a greater number of legislative achievements (Simonton, 1986). Moreover, the success of Machiavellian leaders was significantly enhanced when paired with higher levels of intelligence. In additional to Machiavellianism, narcissism significantly predicted both ratings of the US presidents' charisma and several measures of their performance (Deluga, 1997).

Indeed, narcissism has received outsized attention in this area. Narcissistic CEOs influence organizational performance (Chatterjee & Hambrick, 2007; Resick, Whitman, Weingarden, & Hiller, 2009). These CEOs tend to favor big, bold actions – actions that grab attention. Such actions tend to have large consequences, which can be positive or negative: big wins or big losses (Chatterjee & Hambrick, 2007). Consequently, organizations with narcissistic CEOs tend to perform in an extreme and fluctuating way; their year-to-year performance is less stable than organizations led by less narcissistic CEOs. In addition, highly narcissistic CEOs appear to be less responsive to external cues about their leadership ability than less narcissistic CEOs (Chatterjee & Hambrick, 2011). Finally, narcissistic CEOs are generally compensated more highly and have larger discrepancies in compensation compared to the other executives in their organizations (O'Reilly, Doerr, Caldwell, & Chatman, 2014).

## Managerial Derailment

Research into managerial derailment has suggested that dark personality traits are an important domain to consider in explaining leader failure (Ettner, Maclean, & French, 2011; Hogan & Hogan, 2001; Leslie & Van Velsor, 1996; Lombardo, Ruderman, & McCauley, 1988). One potential reason why individuals attain and maintain leadership positions is that their supervisors tend to ignore moral shortcomings when evaluating managerial potential (Cook & Emmler, 1999; see also Babiak & Hare, 2006 for discussion of specific cases), but what gets you to the top is not necessarily what keeps you there. There are some consistent reasons why executives derail, many of which are highly reminiscent dark personality characteristics, in particular, *problems with interpersonal relationships* (Van Velsor & Leslie, 1995). This domain is consists of interpersonal styles characterized as *insensitive, manipulative, demanding, authoritarian, self-isolating, aloof*, or *critical* (Lombardo & McCauley, 1994), or *arrogance, melodrama, volatility, excessive caution, habitual distrust, aloofness, mischievousness, eccentricity, passive resistance, perfectionism*, and *eagerness to please* (Dotlitch & Cairo, 2003), all of which bear more than a passing resemblance to the HDS or Dark Tetrad dimensions. Especially for areas such as distrust, arrogance, mischievousness, and manipulativeness, which are hallmarks of Dark Tetrad characteristics, we would expect such outcomes: these tactics are likely to produce good short-term outcomes, as discussed above, but to have long-term negative consequences. But other characteristics, such as eccentricity, which is a key feature of schizotypal personality or aloofness, a hallmark of schizoid personality, and melodrama, which might associate with either histrionic or borderline personality, might be ignored in a star performer, but eventually are likely to cause substantial problems as a person's job becomes more about managing others and less about the original technical core was (e.g., Peter & Hull, 1969). We sometimes illustrate this with the example of Michael Scott from the US version of *The Office*: Michael was one of Dunder-Mifflin's best salespeople, which is why he was promoted to management, in spite of many obvious character flaws such as deep levels of insecurity and an inability to understand the feelings of others. To be fair, Michael is probably a mild narcissist, but he is more *dysfunctional* than *dark*.

In contrast to derailment, it is important to examine when dark personality characteristics play a positive role in leaders' careers (Dutton, 2012; cf., Babiak & Hare, 2006; Ghaemi, 2011). For instance, Harms et al. (2011a) primarily framed their study on the role that dark side personality plays in leader development from the perspective of derailment, under the assumption that dark characteristics would generally lead to the sorts of behavior discussed before. Their findings that some dark characteristics, such as narcissism, may accelerate leader development indicate that far more work is needed to determine the functional role that dark personality characteristics play in career advancement and derailment processes. We consider next two extreme cases, narcissism and paranoia. Narcissism is likely to have at least some positive consequences for leader development, whereas paranoia is likely to have negative consequences for development, full stop.

A characteristic like narcissism can hypothetically *drive* development under the right set of circumstances. For instance, Harms et al. (2011a) discuss the example provided by Napoleon, who was not necessarily a bright student, but was a voracious reader of all things related to military strategy. This suggests that narcissists may be motivated to do the work to be the best in an area, at least when that area is important to their self-concepts. On the other hand, a narcissist who did not care about the domain would be likely to avoid putting effort into something that he or she did not care about. Such a state of affairs would lead to generally inconsistent relationships between narcissism and development, since only a subset of narcissists who care about the domain would be so motivated and who would develop fast relative to their low narcissism peers, while the unmotivated narcissists would likely develop slower (or not at all!). This would imply that the trick for developing a narcissistic leader is just getting him or her to care about leadership, to see him or herself as a leader.

In the specific case of career advancement, it makes a great deal of sense that narcissism would play a positive role. In the classic study *Real Managers*, Luthans, Hodgetts, and Rosenkrantz (1988) distinguished between *effective* and *successful* managers. Effective managers lead their teams and get work accomplished. Successful managers get promoted. Effective managers spend most of their time in communication with their teams, while successful managers engage in networking and office politics. Narcissists are good at making first impressions (Paulhus, Westlake, Calvez, & Harms, 2013), so it should be expected that they are good at the activities that lead to managerial success. It is also worth noting that Luthans and colleagues found that only about 10% of managers were both effective *and* successful, suggesting that hard-working managers might benefit from learning a bit of self-promotion from their more narcissistic colleagues (cf., Jonason, Slomski, & Partyka, 2012).

In contrast to narcissism, a characteristic such as paranoia is very likely to serve as a block against development and therefore career advancement. Consider the perception of other people that the paranoid individual has: others are all bad and out to get them. So, when someone offers the paranoid individual advice, encouragement, or correction, this individual is likely to think something along the lines of, "This seems helpful, but you are trying to trick me and undermine me." So, at best, the individual will ignore the advice, and at worst, will actively try to do the opposite.

Intervening to decrease an individual's paranoid tendencies would therefore be very challenging, as it will likely take considerable convincing that you are on the paranoid's side.

## *Incompetent or Evil?*

As we will revisit below, leaders can be a significant source of stress for their followers. This is particularly the case for dysfunctional leaders (e.g., Rose, Shuck, Twyford, & Bergman, 2015). Whether a person's boss is *incompetent* or *malicious*, it is likely to negatively impact that person's well-being. Many of the characteristics we have examined bear on this point. Indeed, it seems natural to consider the relationship between negative aspects of leadership and dark personality (Krasikova, Green, & LeBreton, 2013; Padilla et al., 2007). It has been suggested that the base rate for managerial incompetence in the United States is between 50% and 75% (Hogan, Raskin, & Fazzini, 1990). Moreover, a number of researchers have pointed to dark personality as a key culprit in the ongoing problems with failed leadership in organizations (Burke, 2006; Dotlitch & Cairo, 2003; Hogan, 1994; Kellerman, 2004; Kets de Vries & Miller, 1984).

What are the key differences between managers who are incompetent from managers who are malicious? Krasikova et al. (2013) clarify the differences between ineffective leadership and *destructive* leadership — leadership actions that have intent to cause some form of harm. Krasikova and colleagues highlight a definition of destructive leadership that subsumes various other approaches to "bad" leadership, such as abusive supervision (Tepper, 2000) and petty tyranny (Ashforth, 1994), but excludes *laissez-faire* or absentee leadership, which has been classified as a destructive form of leadership (cf., Skogstad, Einarsen, Torsheim, Aasland, & Hetland, 2007; we discuss this further in terms of employee stress below). Destructive leadership consists of voluntary leader behavior that harms or intends to harm the organization or its members by influencing them to pursue behaviors that are contrary to the organization's legitimate interests or using a leadership style that directly involves harmful methods of influence regardless of the justifications for these behaviors (Krasikova et al., 2013, p. 1310). For instance, a leader may encourage an employee to hide evidence of accounting fraud or illegal waste disposal *in order to protect the organization*, which is a possible form of *unethical pro-organizational behavior* (Umphress & Bingham, 2011). Such a behavior contravenes the organization's legitimate goals, regardless of the fact that the motivations are sincere. A leader may threaten or coerce a subordinate into actions that ensure a bonus or promotion for the leader, a self-serving action on the leader's part that clearly falls within the scope of Krasikova and colleagues' definition (Krasikova et al., 2013; cf., Rose et al., 2015).

Leaders with dispositional characteristics that lead them to impute hostile motives in others (e.g., Skeptical personality, aggressiveness) are more likely to engage in destructive leadership (Krasikova et al., 2013), in part because perceiving hostile motives in others has a tendency to increase the perceived value or justification of aggressive actions in the mind of the actor (Crick & Dodge, 1994). For example, Machiavellian leaders are rated as more abusive by their subordinates than low Machiavellians are (Kiazid, Restubog, Zagenczyk, & Kiewitz, 2010). In a similar vein, charismatic narcissistic leaders can almost be expected to abuse their power (e.g., Sankowsky, 1995). Leaders with psychopathic tendencies can be endlessly destructive, and may be overrepresented in some sectors, such as finance (Babiak & Hare, 2006), where their harmful behaviors can have consequences that extend to people well outside the organization.

Krasikova et al. (2013) model of destructive leadership makes an important distinction worth emphasizing: the difference between destructive intentions and destructive outcomes (Krasikova et al. distinguish between destructive *intentions* and destructive *actions*). Consider for example, the classic narcissist holds motives to improve his or her image of himself or herself through dominance over others (Horowitz et al., 2006; cf., Grijalva & Harms, 2014). That is, the narcissist has a potentially destructive *intention* — to make others feel small, but it will not necessarily result in a negative *outcome*. On the other hand, consider an individual with histrionic tendencies. This person may have no intention to cause harm to others, but the obsessive need for attention they display may be extremely disruptive and lead to negative outcomes.

The above discussion makes it clear that there are at least two ways that a personality characteristic could be labeled "dark" — the underlying nature of the characteristic or in its effects (we have before posited that this distinction underlies the primary difference in focus between the Dark Triad/Tetrad, which is primarily concerned with *motives* or intent, and the HDS which is concerned with typical behavior; Spain et al., 2014). A personality concept is most likely to be labeled *dark* if it has a particularly noxious or malevolent character (Paulhus & Williams, 2002). For instance, a psychopathic boss bullying a submissive employee because the employee annoyed him or her, or an everyday sadist doing the same for the simple thrill of it is clearly acting in a manner we would label *dark* or destructive, and this fits very clearly with the Krasikova et al. (2013) definition.

On the other hand, a characteristic that has no particularly malevolent content could still produce bad consequences. For example, a histrionic boss might demand so much of subordinates' attention that those subordinates find themselves facing severe time pressure to finish their actual job tasks. A schizoid leader may have no motivation to do harm, but the social and emotional distance he or she prefers may leave subordinates with little guidance or support leading to substantial confusion about their job tasks and deadlines (e.g., Skogstand, Hetland, Glasø, & Einarsen, 2014). In both of these cases, the leader's emotional needs (attention and distance, respectively) cause the leader to take actions that lead to substantial role stress for their followers, even though that is not the leader's direct intention. These examples should therefore make clear that bad outcomes can easily arise through either bad intentions or incidentally, and we believe that any discussion of dark characteristics, particularly in their relation to stress and well-being, needs to respect this distinction between intent and effect. That being said, when we consider the role of leader behavior in subordinate stress, the distinction may not be so important, after all. That is, whether your boss is evil or incompetent probably does not matter to you if the boss's behavior is ruining your day.

## LEADERSHIP AND WORK STRESS

### *Leaders as a Source of Stress*

The individual's supervisor is sometimes considered a lens through which the rest of the work experience is viewed (Gerstner & Day, 1997, p. 840). As such, an individual's leader can be a significant factor in their experience of occupational stress, either positively (serving as a protective buffer) or negatively (as a source of stress; Schmidt et al., 2014). As far as protective factors go, it seems fairly clear that transformational leadership serves to buffer the effects of stress (e.g., Lyons & Schneider, 2009; Schmidt et al., 2014; Syrek, Apostel, & Antoni, 2013). In the other direction, the model presented in Fig. 1 illustrates how leader's dark characteristics interact with situational stressors to harm their subordinates' well-being. In general, we expect that the connection between dark characteristics and destructive or dysfunction behavior will be relatively weak, such that the leader's behavior is tolerable under many circumstances. We expect that environmental stressors, such as time pressure or role ambiguity for the leader/team, will typically increase the dysfunctionality or destructiveness of the leader's behavior. Below, however, we primarily focus on the direct dark personality to behavior link, specifically focusing on how leaders' behaviors create stress for their followers.

Sidle (2007) suggests that employees may feel particularly stressed by micromanaging bosses, but that more "hands off" leaders may be a greater problem. In particular, leaders who use a *laissez-faire* (avoidant) style may be a particular source of stress for their subordinates (Skogstad, Hetland, Glasø, & Einarsen, 2014). One highly important stressor that people experience in the workplace is *role ambiguity* – a lack of clarity about what expectations they need to meet (Beehr, 1995). Absentee leaders actively avoid their subordinates and therefore provide the subordinates with little guidance about expectations, likely leading to stress via role ambiguity (Skogstad et al., 2014). In particular, we would expect that Cautious (Avoidant) and Reserved (Schizoid) managers, due to their tendencies toward social and emotional distance, are likely to be absentee managers, leading to greater role ambiguity for their followers.

Other highly stressful experiences might involve the Excitable (Borderline) leader. These leaders take a keen interest in a person or project only to become quickly disillusioned and can also be expected to display considerable emotional instability (see, e.g., Hogan & Hogan, 2009). A follower working for such a leader can only form an expectation that the leader's behavior will be unstable. It may be easier to dismiss a leader who is always unpleasant than one who is sometimes engaged and enthusiastic and other times detached and negative (e.g., Duffy, Ganster, & Pagon, 2002). That is, it takes more emotional resources on the part of the follower to deal with the emotional and relational instability of the Excitable leader than a leader who is consistently unpleasant (Duffy et al., 2002).

## Stressful Situations and Leader Emergence

It has been hypothesized that individuals would prefer a visionary, charismatic leader in times of stress (e.g., Weber, 1947). Halverson, Murphy, and Riggio's (2004) laboratory experiments seem to indicate that this is largely perceptual on the part of followers. Teams in randomly assigned crisis situations rated their randomly assigned leaders as more charismatic than teams not undergoing crises. Oreg and Berson (2015) have found that stressful conditions moderate the relationship between approach-oriented personality traits (extraversion and openness to experience) and leader charisma. These personality characteristics show positive relationships with charisma under low stress conditions, but the relationships flatten out under high stress.

That said, we might expect stress to induce differential effects on different dimensions of the Dark Tetrad. For example, some research has shown a positive relationship between narcissism and charismatic leadership (e.g., Sankowsky, 1995), but it is likely that the nastier aspects of narcissism will tend to leak out when their egos are threatened by the potential for loss. However, we also know that followers tend to prefer leaders in a crisis who can project a sense of confidence and who promises to provide a path forward in order to end the stressful situation. Narcissists are likely to attempt to fill this role.

In terms of other dark traits, we could imagine that leaders characterized by higher levels of psychopathy will be relatively unresponsive to stressful situations because they tend not to experience fear or emotions in general. Machiavellianism might be even more complicated in that it is possible that a skilled Machiavellian would attempt to take advantage of stressful, crisis situations to gain a leadership position. A popular illustration of this latter point can be drawn from the Netflix drama *House of Cards*, in which Frank Underwood manipulates events, and more importantly, other people's emotional and strategic responses to those events, to assume the US presidency without being elected to the office. Underwood is a clear illustration of a character high in both Machiavellianism and psychopathy.

# DARK PERSONALITY CHARACTERISTICS AND THE EXPERIENCE OF STRESS

In general, we can study how personality characteristics moderate the impact of events on people's reactions to those events. This is the role that personality characteristics play in Affective Events Theory (Weiss & Cropanzano, 1996), for instance. An individual experiences some event at work and interprets that event in a personality-dependent way. As an example, a Skeptical person, who distrusts others as a rule, may interpret a request from a coworker for feedback on that coworker's performance as a kind of trap, "Ah, I see, you are trying to get me to criticize you so that you can complain about me to our boss!" and therefore feel threatened, motivating him or her to provide dishonest feedback. A less skeptical person would likely take the experience at face value, feeling either neutral or perhaps somewhat positive about being valued enough to be asked for feedback. These negative versus positive interpretations of events influence the individual's view of the organization and their work situation over time. Similarly, in the stress-strain relationship, personality characteristics often serve as moderators. For instance, an internal locus of control (Rotter, 1966) provides a buffer against strain under the experience of stress (e.g., Kahn & Byosiere, 1992). There is little reason to believe that dark side personality is fundamentally different, though there are some important distinctions to discuss before we move on.

For instance, individuals with different dark personality characteristics should be expected to respond to stressful situations differently from one another. We might suppose that vulnerable narcissists might, under the weight of their inflated but fragile egos, crumble in the face of pressure, while the grandiose narcissists might simply laugh it off as inconsequential, since they are so great anyway. The evidence does not seem to bear this out: narcissists, in general, produce more stress hormones in response to negative circumstances (Cheng, Tracy, & Miller, 2013). In addition, psychopaths also show increased emotional reactivity to stressful conditions compared those lower in psychopathy (Noser, Zeigler-Hill, & Besser, 2014). However, there is some evidence that dark characteristics might have direct impact on well-being. Specifically, narcissists may have higher well-being than non-narcissists (Hill & Roberts, 2012), at least in adolescence and early adulthood, though such findings do not appear to apply throughout the lifespan.

Above, we discussed the difference in emphasis between the Dark Tetrad approach and the HDS approach. The Dark Triad is more about an individual's social motives, whereas the HDS is more about the individual's interpersonal style under some circumstances. Each of these conceptualizations has different implications for the role that dark personality plays in the stress process. For one, the Dark Tetrad very naturally aligns with the individual as a source of stress for others, whereas the HDS implies that a person's dark characteristics will become most damaging to their well-being when they are under high stress. Of course there are other considerations, but these implications stand out.

### An Unfolding Model of Dark Personality, Stress, and Leadership

We propose a downward spiral for dark personality characteristics and stress. As discussed above, there is reason to suspect that dark personality characteristics, at least under the HDS conception, are *beneficial* at least some of the time. Additionally, the Dark Triad/Tetrad perspective to some extent also emphasizes effective short-term strategies that have negative long-term effects. Under considerable stress, however, the behaviors associated with these characteristics can become damaging, potentially even in the short term. We will consider narcissism as our key example because it is probably the best-understood of the dark personality characteristics (Grijalva & Harms, 2014; Spain et al., 2014).

We begin our example by thinking of our hypothetical narcissist's first day at work, ignoring the fact that they were already probably more likely to get hired due to their self-enhancing style in interviews (Paulhus et al., 2013). They engage in a variety of soft and hard influence tactics to get their goals accomplished (Jonason et al., 2012). They engage in self-promotion and self-enhancement when interacting with anyone hierarchically above them, but are often domineering toward those hierarchically beneath them (e.g., Babiak & Hare, 2006; Grijalva & Harms, 2014; cf., Spain et al., 2014). They may even work hard to be highly competent and recognized for this competence (Harms et al., 2011a). This combination typically leads to success (Luthans et al., 1988), and does so in this case. Eventually, the narcissist is promoted to a level where his or her difficulty maintaining social relationships and disdain for others leads to poor relationships with peers and subordinates, though they may still be well-regarded by higher management (Babiak & Hare, 2006 provide numerous examples). At this point, if the narcissist is sufficiently strong and charismatic, they may still be able to get subordinates to play into their self-serving agenda, but if not they may face a rebellion that diminishes their power (Sankowsky, 1995). If this happens additional shocks could derail the individual's career.

Even for the successful narcissist, the position illustrated above is difficult. Their behavior has made them increasingly distant from the social resources they need to continue doing an effective job, and these resources become more and more important as their career progresses. The socially isolated narcissist is increasingly vulnerable to random circumstances (cf., Vroom & MacCrimmons, 1968). That is, with fewer resources to draw on, they are increasingly likely to fail when unexpected circumstances happen, diminishing their reputation, which is the main resource they still possess. Enough such circumstances and their career will likely to derail.

# CONCLUSION

The study of dark personality is essentially as old as psychology itself. Recent scandals in the corporate world have fueled heightened interest in these characteristics in the organizational sciences. We have attempted to provide a thorough, but compact guide to the large and complicated domain of dark personality characteristics, paying special attention to the roles that they play in leadership and the stress process. While thorough, our review is far from comprehensive, there are vast swaths of the literature that do not fit comfortably in this space, but our review should provide adequate pointers.

There are several approaches to assessing the dark side of personality, but they all imply that the most malignant forms involve harming and dominating others, thus the Dark Triad/Tetrad warrants understanding from this point-of-view. The also agree that these characteristics can provide advantages under some circumstances, but harm under others. We believe that these characteristics are extremely important for understanding employee development and career advancement; in particular, being aware of the self-serving and self-enhancing tactics used by "dark" individuals is important for balancing effectiveness and success in managers. Finally, understanding the role that these characteristics play in stress experiences at work is extremely important, especially since bad leaders can cause so much suffering for their subordinates.

# REFERENCES

Ajzen, I. (1991). The theory of planned behavior. *Organizational Behavior and Human Decision Processes*, *50*, 179−211.

American Psychological Association. (1994). *Diagnostic and statistical manual of mental disorders* (4th ed.). Washington, DC: American Psychological Association.

Antonakis, J., Day, D. V., & Schyns, B. (2012). Leadership and individual differences: At the cusp of a renaissance. *The Leadership Quarterly*, *23*, 643−650.

Ashforth, B. E. (1994). Petty tyranny in organizations. *Human Relations*, *47*, 755−778.

Ashton, M., Lee, K., Perugini, M., Szarota, P., de Vries, R., Di Blas, L., Boies, K., & De Raad, B. (2004). A six-factor structure of personality-descriptive adjectives: Solutions from psycholexical studies in seven languages. *Journal of Personality and Social Psychology*, *86*, 356−366.

Babiak, P., & Hare, R. (2006). *Snakes in suits: When psychopaths go to work*. New York, NY: Regan Books.

Beehr, T. A. (1995). *Psychological stress in the workplace*. London: Routledge.

Benson, M., & Campbell, J. (2007). To be, or not to be, linear: An expanded representation of personality and its relationship to leadership performance. *International Journal of Selection and Assessment, 15*, 232–249.

Buckels, E. E., Jones, D. N., & Paulhus, D. (2013). Behavioral confirmation of everyday sadism. *Psychological Science, 24*, 2201–2209.

Burke, R. (2006). Why leaders fail: Exploring the darkside. *International Journal of Manpower, 27*, 91–100.

Campbell, W. K., Hoffman, B. J., Campbell, S. M., & Marchiso, G. (2011). Narcissism in organizational contexts. *Human Resource Management Review, 21*, 268–284.

Chatterjee, A., & Hambrick, D. C. (2007). It's all about me: Narcissistic chief executive officers and their effects on company strategy and performance. *Administrative Science Quarterly, 52*, 351–386.

Chatterjee, A., & Hambrick, D. C. (2011). Executive personality, capability cues, and risk-taking: How narcissistic CEOs react to their successes and stumbles. *Administrative Science Quarterly, 56*, 202–237.

Cheng, J. T., Tracy, J. L., & Miller, G. E. (2013). Are narcissists hardy or vulnerable? The role of narcissism in the production of stress-related biomarkers in response to emotional distress. *Emotion, 13*, 1004–1011.

Christie, R., & Geis, F. L. (1970). *Studies in Machiavellianism.* New York, NY: Academic Press.

Cleckley, H. (1976). *The mask of sanity* (5th ed.). St. Louis, MO: Mosby.

Cook, T., & Emmler, N. (1999). Bottom up versus top down evaluations of candidates' managerial potential: An experimental study. *Journal of Occupational and Organizational Psychology, 72*, 423–440.

Crick, N. R., & Dodge, K. A. (1994). A review and reformulation of social information-processing mechanisms in children's social adjustment. *Psychological Bulletin, 115*, 74–101.

Deluga, R. (2001). American presidential Machiavellianism: Implications for charismatic leadership and rated performance. *The Leadership Quarterly, 12*, 339–363.

Deluga, R. J. (1997). Relationship among American presidential charismatic leadership, narcissism, and rated performance. *The Leadership Quarterly, 8*(1), 49–65.

Digman, J. M. (1990). Personality structure: Emergence of the five-factor model. *Annual Review of Psychology, 41*, 417–440.

Dotlitch, D., & Cairo, P. (2003). *Why CEOs fail: The 11 behaviors that can derail your climb to the top and how to manage them.* San Francisco, CA: Jossey-Bass.

Duffy, M. K., Ganster, D. C., & Pagon, M. (2002). Social undermining in the workplace. *Academy of Management Journal, 45*, 331–351.

Dutton, K. (2012). *The wisdom of psychopaths: What saints, spies, and serial killers can teach us about success.* New York, NY: Scientific American.

Ettner, S., Maclean, S. C., & French, M. (2011). Does having a dysfunctional personality hurt your career? Axis II personality disorders and labor market outcomes. *Industrial Relations, 50*, 149–173.

Gerstner, C. R., & Day, D. V. (1997). Meta-analytic review of leader-member exchange theory: Correlates and construct issues. *Journal of Applied Psychology, 82*, 827–844.

Ghaemi, N. (2011). *A first-rate madness.* New York, NY: The Penguin Press.

Gintis, H. (2007). A framework for the unification of the behavioral sciences. *Behavioral and Brain Sciences, 30*, 1–61.

Goldberg, L. (1993). The structure of phenotypic personality traits. *American Psychologist,* *48,* 26–34.

Grijalva, E., & Harms, P. D. (2014). Narcissism: An integrative synthesis and dominance-complementarity model. *Academy of Management Perspectives, 28,* 108–127.

Grijalva, E., Harms, P. D., Newman, D., Gaddis, B., & Fraley, R. C. (2015). Narcissism and leadership: A meta-analytic review of linear and nonlinear relationships. *Personnel Psychology, 68,* 1–47.

Guenole, N. (2014). Maladaptive personality at work: Exploring the darkness. *Industrial and Organizational Psychology: Perspectives on Science and Practice, 7,* 85–97.

Halverson, S. K., Murphy, S. E., & Riggio, R. E. (2004). Charismatic leadership in crisis situations: A laboratory investigation of stress and crisis. *Small Group Research, 35,* 495–514.

Hare, R. D. (1985). Checklist for the assessment of psychopathy in criminal populations. In M. H. Ben-Aron, S. J. Hucker, & C. D. Webster (Eds.), *Clinical criminology* (pp. 157–167). University of Toronto, ON: Clarke Institute of Psychiatry.

Hare, R. D. (1999). *Without conscience: The disturbing world of the psychopaths among us.* New York, NY: Guilford Press.

Harms, P. D., & Spain, S. M. (2015). Beyond the bright side: Dark personality at work. *Applied Psychology: An International Review, 64,* 15–24.

Harms, P. D., Spain, S. M., & Hannah, S. T. (2011a). Leader development and the dark side of personality. *The Leadership Quarterly, 22,* 495–509.

Harms, P. D., Spain, S. M., Hannah, S. T., Hogan, J., & Foster, J. W. (2011b). You underestimate the power of the dark side: Subclinical traits, the big 5, and performance. Paper presented at the Society for Industrial and Organizational Psychology annual conference, Chicago, IL.

Harms, P. D., Spain, S. M., & Wood, D. (2014). Mapping personality in dark places. *Industrial and Organizational Psychology: Perspectives on Science and Practice, 7,* 114–117.

Harms, P. D., Wood, D., & Spain, S. (2016). Separating the why from the what: A reply to Jonas and Markon. *Psychological Review, 123,* 84–89.

Hill, P. L., & Roberts, B. W. (2012). Narcissism, well-being, and observer-rated personality across the lifespan. *Social Psychological and Personality Science, 3,* 216–223.

Hiller, N., DeChurch, L., Murase, T., & Doty, D. (2011). Searching for outcomes of leadership: A 25-year review. *Journal of Management, 37,* 1137–1177.

Hogan, R. (1994). Trouble at the top: Causes and consequences of managerial incompetence. *Consulting Psychology Journal, 46,* 9–15.

Hogan, R. (2007). *Personality and the fate of organizations.* Mahwah, NJ: Lawrence Erlbaum Associates, Inc.

Hogan, R., & Hogan, J. (2001). Assessing leadership: A view from the dark side. *International Journal of Selection and Assessment, 9,* 40–51.

Hogan, R., & Hogan, J. (2009). *Hogan development survey manual* (3rd ed.). Tulsa, OK: Hogan Assessment Systems.

Hogan, R., & Kaiser, R. (2005). What we know about leadership. *Review of General Psychology, 9,* 169–180.

Hogan, R., Raskin, R., & Fazzini, D. (1990). The dark side of charisma. In K. E. Clark (Eds.) *Measures of leadership* (pp. 343–354). West Orange, NJ: Leadership Library of America.

Horowitz, L. J., Wilson, K. R., Turan, B., Zolotsev, P., Constantino, M. J., & Henderson, L. (2006). How interpersonal motives clarify the meaning of interpersonal behavior: A revised circumplex model. *Personality and Social Psychology Review, 10*, 67–86.

Johnson, D., Wrangham, R., & Rosen, S. (2002). Is military incompetence adaptive? An empirical test with risk-taking behavior in modern warfare. *Evolution and Human Behavior, 23*, 245–264.

Jonason, P. K., Koenig, B., & Tost, J. (2010). Living a fast life: The Dark Triad and life history theory. *Human Nature, 21*, 428–442.

Jonason, P. K., Slomski, S., & Partyka, J. (2012). The dark triad at work: How toxic employees get their way. *Personality and Individual Differences, 52*, 449–453.

Jonason, P. K., & Webster, G. D. (2010). The dirty dozen: A concise measure of the Dark Triad. *Psychological Assessment, 22*, 420–432.

Jones, D. N., & Paulhus, D. L. (2009). Machiavellianism. In M. R. Leary & R. H. Hoyle (Eds.). *Handbook of individual differences in social behavior* (pp. 93–108). New York, NY: Guilford.

Judge, T. A., Piccolo, R., & Kosalka, T. (2009). The bright side and dark side of leader traits: A review and theoretical extension of the leader trait paradigm. *The Leadership Quarterly, 20*, 855–875.

Kahn, R. L., & Byosiere, P. (1992). Stress in organizations. In M. Dunnette & L. Hough (Eds.), *Handbook of industrial and organizational psychology* (2nd ed., Vol. 3, pp. 571–650). Palo Alto, CA: Consulting Psychologist Press.

Kellerman, B. (2004). *Bad leadership: What it is, how it happens, why it matters*. Boston, MA: Harvard Business School Publishing.

Kets de Vries, M., & Miller, D. (1984). Neurotic style and organizational pathology. *Strategic Management Journal, 5*, 35–55.

Kets de Vries, M., & Miller, D. (1985). Narcissism and leadership: An object relations perspective. *Human Relations, 38*, 583–601.

Kiazid, K., Restubog, S., Zagenczyk, T., & Kiewitz, C. (2010). In pursuit of power: The role of authoritarian leadership in the relationship between supervisors' Machiavellianism and subordinates' perceptions of abusive supervisory behavior. *Journal of Research in Personality, 44*, 512–519.

Krasikova, D., Green, S. G., & LeBreton, J. L. (2013). Destructive leadership: A theoretical review, integration, and future research agenda. *Journal of Management, 39*, 1308–1338.

LeBreton, J. M., Binning, J. F., & Adorno, A. J. (2006). Subclinical psychopaths. In J. C. Thomas & D. Segal (Eds.), *Comprehensive handbook of personality and psychopathology personality and everyday functioning* (Vol. I, pp. 388–411). New York, NY: Wiley.

Lee, K., & Ashton, M. (2005). Psychopathy, Machiavellianism, and narcissism in the five-factor model and the HEXACO model of personality structure. *Personality and Individual Differences, 38*, 1571–1582.

Leslie, J., & Van Velsor, E. (1996). *A look at derailment today: North America and Europe*. Greensboro, NC: Center for Creative Leadership.

Lombardo, M., & McCauley, C. (1994). *Benchmarks: A manual and trainer's guide*. Greensboro, NC: Center for Creative Leadership.

Lombardo, M., Ruderman, M., & McCauley, C. (1988). Explanations of success and derailment in upper-level management positions. *Journal of Business and Psychology, 2*, 199–216.

Luthans, F., Hodgetts, R. M., & Rosenkrantz, S. A. (1988). *Real managers*. Cambridge, MA: Ballinger Publishing Co.

Lyons, J. B., & Schneider, T. R. (2009). The effects of leadership style on stress outcomes. *The Leadership Quarterly, 20*, 737–748.

McCrae, R., & Costa, P. (1995). Trait explanations in personality psychology. *European Journal of Personality, 9*, 231–252.

Miller, J., Gentile, B., Wilson, L., & Campbell, W. K. (2013). Grandiose and vulnerable narcissism and the DSM-5 pathological personality trait model. *Journal of Personality Assessment, 95*, 284–290.

Morf, C. C., & Rhodewalt, F. (2001). Unraveling the paradoxes of narcissism: A dynamic self-regulatory processing model. *Psychological Inquiry, 12*, 177–196.

Noser, A. E., Zeigler-Hill, V., & Besser, A. (2014). Stress and affective experiences: The importance of dark personality features. *Journal of Research in Personality, 53*, 158–164.

O'Boyle, E. H., Forsyth, D. R., Banks, G. C., & McDaniel, M. A. (2012). A meta-analysis of the dark triad and work behavior: A social exchange perspective. *Journal of Applied Psychology, 97*, 557–579.

O'Reilly, C. A., Jr., Doerr, B., Caldwell, D. F., & Chatman, J. A. (2014). Narcissistic CEOs and executive compensation. *The Leadership Quarterly, 25*, 218–231.

Oreg, S., & Berson, Y. (2015). Personality and charismatic leadership: The moderating role of situational stress. *Personnel Psychology, 68*, 49–77.

Padilla, A., Hogan, R., & Kaiser, R. B. (2007). The toxic triangle: Destructive leaders, susceptible followers, and conducive environments. *The Leadership Quarterly, 18*, 176–194.

Paulhus, D. (2014). Toward a taxonomy of dark personalities. *Current Directions in Psychological Science, 23*, 421–426.

Paulhus, D. L., Westlake, B. G., Calvez, S. S., & Harms, P. D. (2013). Self-presentation style in job interviews: The role of personality and culture. *Journal of Applied Social Psychology, 43*, 2042–2059.

Paulhus, D. L., & Williams, K. (2002). The dark triad of personality: Narcissism, Machiavellianism, and psychopathy. *Journal of Research in Personality, 36*, 556–568.

Peter, L. J., & Hull, R. (1969). *The Peter principle: Why things always go wrong* (1st ed.). New York, NY: HarperCollins.

Raskin, R., & Hall, C. S. (1979). A narcissistic personality inventory. *Psychological Reports, 45*, 590.

Raskin, R., Novacek, J., & Hogan, R. (1991). Narcissism, self-esteem, and defensive self-enhancement. *Journal of Personality, 59*, 19–38.

Resick, C., Whitman, D., Weingarden, S., & Hiller, N. (2009). The bright-side and dark-side of CEO personality: Examining core self-evaluations, narcissism, transformational leadership, and strategic influence. *Journal of Applied Psychology, 94*, 1365–1381.

Roberts, B. W. (2005). Blessings, banes, and possibilities in the study of childhood personality. *Merrill-Palmer Quarterly, 51*, 367–378.

Rose, K., Shuck, B., Twyford, D., & Bergman, M. (2015). Skunked: An integrative review exploring the consequences of the dysfunctional leader and implications for those who work for them. *Human Resource Development Review, 14*, 64–90.

Rosenthal, S. A., & Pittinsky, T. L. (2006). Narcissistic leadership. *The Leadership Quarterly, 17*, 617–633.

Rotter, J. B. (1966). Generalized expectancies for internal versus external control of reinforcement. *Psychological Monographs, 80*(1), 1–28.

Sankowsky, D. (1995). The charismatic leader as narcissist: Understanding the abuse of power. *Organizational Dynamics, 23*, 57–71.

Schmidt, B., Loerbroks, A., Herr, R., Litaker, D., Wilson, M., Kastner, M., & Fischer, J. (2014). Psychosocial resources and the relationship between transformational leadership and employees' psychological strain. *Work, 49*, 315–324.

Sidle, S. D. (2007). The danger of do nothing leaders. *Academy of Management Perspectives, 21*, 75–77. doi:10.5465/AMP.2007.25356514

Simonton, D. (1986). Presidential personality: Biographical use of the Gough adjective checklist. *Journal of Personality and Social Psychology, 51*, 149–160.

Skeem, J., Polaschek, D., Patrick, C., & Lilienfeld, S. (2011). Psychopathic personality: Bridging the gap between scientific evidence and public policy. *Psychological Science in the Public Interest, 12*, 95–162.

Skogstad, A., Einarsen, S., Torsheim, T., Aasland, M. S., & Hetland, H. (2007). The destructiveness of laissez-faire leadership behavior. *Journal of Occupational Health Psychology, 12*, 80–92.

Skogstand, A., Hetland, J., Glasø, L., & Einarsen, S. (2014). Is avoidant leadership a root cause of subordinate stress? Longitudinal relationships between laissez-faire leadership and role ambiguity. *Work and Stress, 28*, 323–341. doi:10.1037/t03624-000

Spain, S. M., Harms, P. D., & LeBreton, J. M. (2014). The dark side of personality at work. *Journal of Organizational Behavior, 35*, S41–S60.

Syrek, C. J., Apostel, E., & Antoni, C. H. (2013). Stress in highly demanding IT jobs: Transformational leadership moderates the impact of time pressure on exhaustion and work-life balance. *Journal of Occupational Health Psychology, 18*, 252–261.

Tepper, B. J. (2000). Consequences of abusive supervision. *Academy of Management Journal, 43*, 178–190.

Umphress, E., & Bingham, J. (2011). When employees do bad things for good reasons: Examining unethical pro-organizational behaviors. *Organizational Science, 22*, 621–640.

Van Velsor, E., & Leslie, J. B. (1995). Why executives derail: Perspectives across time and cultures. *Academy of Management Executive, 9*, 62–72.

Vroom, V., & MacCrimmon, K. R. (1968). Toward a stochastic theory of managerial careers. *Administrative Science Quarterly, 13*, 26–46.

Weber, M. (1947). *The theory of social and economic organizations* (T. Parsons, Trans.). New York, NY: Free Press.

Weiss, H. M., & Cropanzano, R. (1996). Affective events theory: A theoretical discussion of the structure, causes, and consequences of affective experiences at work. In B. M. Staw & L. L. Cummings (Eds.), *Research in organizational behavior* (Vol. 18, pp. 1–74). Greenwich, CT: JAI Press.

Wiggins, J. S. (1996). *The five-factor model of personality: Theoretical perspectives*. New York, NY: Guilford.

Wood, D., Gardner, M. H., & Harms, P. D. (2015). How functionalist and process approaches to behavior can explain trait covariation. *Psychological Review, 122*, 84–111. doi:10.1037/a0038423

Wu, J., & LeBreton, J. M. (2011). Reconsidering the dispositional basis of counterproductive work behavior: The role of aberrant personality traits. *Personnel Psychology, 64*, 593–626.

Zaccaro, S. (2012). Individual differences and leadership: Contributions to a third tipping point. *The Leadership Quarterly, 23*, 718–728.

# THE PROMISE AND PERIL OF WORKPLACE CONNECTIONS: INSIGHTS FOR LEADERS ABOUT WORKPLACE NETWORKS AND WELL-BEING

Kristin L. Cullen-Lester, Alexandra Gerbasi and Sean White

## ABSTRACT

*This chapter utilizes a network perspective to show how the totality of one's social connections impacts well-being by providing access to resources (e.g., information, feedback, and support) and placing limits on autonomy. We provide a brief review of basic network concepts and explain the importance of understanding how the networks in which leaders are embedded may enhance or diminish their well-being. Further, with this greater understanding, we describe how leaders can help promote the well-being of their employees. In particular, we focus on four key aspects of workplace networks that are likely to impact well-being: centrality, structural holes, embeddedness, and negative ties. We not*

The Role of Leadership in Occupational Stress
Research in Occupational Stress and Well Being, Volume 14, 61–90
Copyright © 2016 by Emerald Group Publishing Limited
All rights of reproduction in any form reserved
ISSN: 1479-3555/doi:10.1108/S1479-355520160000014003

*only discuss practical implications for leaders' well-being and the well-being of their employees, but also suggest directions for future research.*

**Keywords:** Social networks; well-being; centrality; structural holes; negative ties; energy

The interaction and interdependence employees have with coworkers and customers have increased with the shift from a manufacturing to a service and knowledge economy (Griffin, Neal, & Parker, 2007). Many organizations have flattened their structures in an attempt to improve collaboration, including adopting matrix and team-based organizational designs (Ilgen, Hollenbeck, Johnson, & Jundt, 2005; Strikwerda & Stoelhorst, 2009). Technological advancements (e.g., collaboration technologies, mobile devices, social networking apps, texting, video conferencing) are commonly used to allow for dynamic, interdependent interaction between workers locally, across the globe, and beyond traditional work hours (Butts, Becker, & Boswell, 2015; Dean & Webb, 2011). These changes have made workplace relationships a vital and pervasive part of work life (Borgatti & Cross, 2003; Grant & Parker, 2009).

In many ways, relationships have the potential to enrich employees' work experience by stimulating positive emotions and promoting their well-being, but they also have the potential to elicit negative emotions and undermine employees' well-being. Indeed, relationships have been identified as one of the most common sources of work stress, especially when they fail to provide the social support employees need or when they are harmful (i.e., sources of hostility, aggression, or violence; Sauter, Murphy, & Hurrell, 1990). Although, individual relationships are clearly important for well-being, this chapter utilizes a network perspective to show how the totality of one's social connections impacts well-being by providing access to resources (e.g., information, feedback, and support) and placing limits on autonomy.

The management literature has increasingly recognized the importance of the networks, in which employees are embedded, for individual, team, and organizational success (e.g., Burt, 1992; Oh, Chung, & Labianca, 2004; Reagans, Zuckerman, & McEvily, 2004). In particular, emerging research points to critical importance of networks for leaders (for a recent review, see Carter, DeChurch, Braun, & Contractor, 2015). Not only do individuals obtain leadership positions because of their social connections, their effectiveness is in part determined by their ability to understand the informal social structure of the workplace, make connections to central people, and facilitate connections between disconnected employees (Brass & Krackhardt, 2012). Effective leaders are posited to accurately perceive their own and the broader social connections within the organization (Balkundi & Kilduff, 2006). Growing research is demonstrating the importance of a leader's network position for their own and collective outcomes. For example, groups whose leaders occupy central and brokering positions tend to perform better (Balkundi & Harrison, 2006; Mehra, Dixon, Brass, & Robertson, 2006).

Emerging research suggests networks are not only beneficial from an instrumental perspective, but also provide affective benefits and have potential costs. The literature examining well-being has traditionally examined the dyadic relationships in which individuals participate as sources of stress, as well as buffers to stress and sources of well-being in their own right (cf. Kawachi & Berkman, 2001). However, this focus does not consider the impact that one's indirect connections can have on well-being. For example, Fowler and Christakis (2008) found that an individual's happiness was influenced by the happiness of people as many as three connections away from them in the network. Other studies have documented the "ripple effects" of affect spreading through a network (Barsade, 2002) as people observe and react to the emotions of those to whom they are connected. For example, Totterdell, Wall, Holman, Diamond, and Epitropaki (2004) found that people who work together have similar work-related affect and that negative affect appeared to be contagious.

Many of the structural changes and technological advancements adopted by organizations to improve collaboration unintentionally overload employees, especially those who occupy critical positions in workplace communication networks (Cross & Gray, 2013). Beyond the sheer numbers of relationships employees have to manage, many employees are expected to "be connected all the time," and are subjected to a continuous stream of information, which has taken a toll, leaving them feeling overwhelmed (Dean & Webb, 2011). In the face of increasingly collaborative demands organizations are concerned about the well-being of their employees. For example, 65% of executives responding to a recent survey reported that employees who are overwhelmed by information and activity is an important or urgent issue for their organization, while 44% said their organization is not ready to address the issue (Global Human Capital Trends, 2014). Collaborative overload is a challenge for many employees, but especially for individuals in formal leadership positions (Balkundi & Kilduff,

2006; Cross & Cummings, 2004). Thus, it is important for leaders to understand how the networks in which they are embedded may be enhancing or diminishing their own well-being. Leaders can also use this knowledge to help promote the well-being of their employees. In the remainder of this chapter, we provide a brief introduction to networks before providing a deeper look at four key aspects of workplace networks that are likely to enhance or diminish well-being. We conclude by discussing practical implications for leaders own well-being and the well-being of their employees and future directions for research.

# RELATIONSHIPS AND EMPLOYEE WELL-BEING

Scholars have long recognized that relationships are central to individuals' experience of stress and well-being (Diener, Suh, Lucas & Smith, 1999; Myers, 2000). Individuals receive affection, confirmation, respect, and status from their social connections and the fit they feel with their social surroundings (Diener, Tay, & Meyers, 2011; Stevenrink & Lindenberg, 2006). The extent to which individuals have meaningful, close relationships with family and friends influences their evaluations of their own life (Myers, 2000). Social support (provided by individuals' relationships) is thought to have a direct beneficial effect on their well-being and to help individuals respond effectively to the stressors they experience (Heaney & Israel, 2008). As such, the relationships in which individuals are embedded are very influential for building or destroying their sense of well-being (Helliwell & Putnam, 2004). The importance of supportive relationships for experiencing positive feelings and having a positive view of one's life has been demonstrated globally across a number of demographic groups (Diener, Ng, Harter, & Arora, 2010; Tay & Diener, 2011). Well-being is a broad subjective evaluation spanning multiple domains, including satisfaction with important aspect of life such as work, as well as the experience positive affect and low levels of negative affect (i.e., moods and emotions; Diener, 2000; Diener et al., 1999). As such, we focus broadly on aspects of well-being related to employees' workplace social environment.

## Positive Workplace Relationships

Positive organizational scholars have examined ways that workplace relationships fulfill employees' affective needs, fuel motivation (Quinn,

Spreitzer, & Lam, 2012), engagement (Clifton & Harter, 2003), satisfaction and well-being (Dutton, 2003). They have also studied how relationships contribute to individual growth and development (Dutton, 2003; Dutton & Heaphy, 2003). Here we review how positive relationships enhance employee well-being by providing support and meaning, transferring energy, and facilitating learning and the experience of vitality.

As with the broader literature, the historical, predominant focus on the driving connection between relationships and well-being in the workplace has been the provision of social support. Indeed, the support received from coworkers and supervisors influences employees' ability to complete their work and their overall experience of the workplace. Previous research has found that employees who do not form meaningful relationships with their supervisor and coworkers have lower job satisfaction (Eisenberger, Stinglhamber, Vandenberghe, Sucharski, & Rhoades, 2002). A meta-analysis found that social support is related to many positive workplace outcomes and acts as a buffer from workplace stressors (Humphrey, Nahrgang & Morgeson, 2007).

Workplace connections can also provide employees with a sense of meaningfulness (Rosso, Dekas, & Wrzesniewski, 2010). One way individuals gain meaningfulness is by giving to others. Giving enhances feelings of self-efficacy (Mogilner, Chance, & Norton, 2012), helps the giver to feel valued (see Blau, 1964) and to see the contribution or impact he/she is making (Grant, 2007, 2012). The giver is also likely to experience gratitude themselves (because they have an opportunity to make a difference) and from others for their actions (Grant & Dutton, 2012). The act of giving improves mental and physical well-being (Grant & Dutton, 2012). Further, giving to others (even more than receiving; Dunn, Aknin, & Norton, 2008) has been found to increase the giver's happiness (Taylor & Turner, 2001). Individuals who have a sense of meaning are more attentive and responsive to others when doing their work (Edmondson, 1999). Employees are more committed, pro-socially motivated, and likely to help others when they understand how their job impacts the well-being of others and have frequent contact with their beneficiaries (Grant, 2007; Grant & Parker, 2009).

Energy is one of the most fundamental resources for performance, health, and well-being at work (Quinn et al., 2012). The level of energy employees experience is influenced by their interactions with others; exchanges that result in positive outcomes lead to the creation of relational energy (Lawler & Yoon, 1993, 1996). Baker, Cross, and Wooten (2003) introduced the term energizing relationships to describe connections that generate positive energy in the workplace. Quinn and Dutton (2005) explain that more than information is exchanged as individuals communicate to organize and align the activities needed to complete shared work. Energy is generated and depleted in these conversations and to what extent this occurs, in part determines the success of the coordination process (Quinn et al., 2012). People who have energizing relationships experience a positive mood that enables them to make a contribution to the organization (Quinn & Dutton, 2005); positive experiences carryover into subsequent interactions, resulting in positive spillover effects (Baker et al., 2003).

An employees' workplace social environment is also thought to have a large impact on employees' thriving; their joint experience of vitality (feeling alive) and learning (sense of improving; Spreitzer, Sutcliffe, Dutton, Sonenshein, & Grant, 2005). As mentioned previously, as people interact, energy and enthusiasm is transferred, impacting mood. Exchanges with others also provide opportunities for learning and having one's thinking challenged and advanced. Recent research has found that positive informal ties lead to higher thriving, job satisfaction, and organizational commitment (Parker, Gerbasi, & Porath, 2013). Thriving helps individuals develop, perform better, reduce strain, and improve their health (Porath, Spreitzer, Gibson, & Garnett, 2012). Whereas negative relationships may be a last straw for someone who is languishing, a thriving individual is better able to withstand negative interactions because they have more personal resources to draw upon (Porath et al., 2012). Thriving employees see themselves on a positive trajectory and learn from others at work regardless of whether their interactions are positive or negative. Those who enjoy a higher state of thriving are likely to be more resilient (Spreitzer, Porath, & Gibson, 2012).

## Networks and Well-Being

As just described, much of the literature linking relationships and well-being has focused on the importance of positive relationships that provide social support, meaning, energy, and opportunities to learn. However, these dyadic connections are the building blocks of larger networks, which also likely impact employees' well-being. By only considering what isolated dyadic relationships provide, we fail to gain insight into how the network in which individuals are embedded can enhance or diminish their well-being. The position individuals have in workplace networks determines the resources and support available to them and can also place them at risk of experiencing greater strain. Further, the structure of the network surrounding individuals constrains their actions and determines the extent to which they are exposed to the flows being transferred between network connections as such an individual's well-being is influenced by not only their connections, but the connections of the people to whom they are connected. Finally, the majority of organizational research has examined positive networks in which individuals would likely benefit from participating (until they are overloaded), but an emerging area of research is examining less desirable workplace networks and their effects on employees' well-being.

In their simplest form, networks consist of a set of nodes and the ties that represent relationships between them (Brass, Galaskiewicz, Greve, & Tsai, 2004). The literature reviewed in this chapter is concerned with studies that have examined people as nodes, but nodes can also be groups, organizations, or other objects. Ties between nodes arise for many different reasons, but are generally social-based (friendship, family bonds), similarity-based (membership in the same group, physical proximity, sharing a trait), interaction-based (talks with, orders from, gives advice to), or information-flow-based (dissemination of ideas or beliefs, political influence) (Borgatti, Everett, & Johnson, 2013). Of course, often multiple types of relationships develop between individuals, constituting what is called a "multiplex" tie.

The type of relationship composing a network is important for understanding the effects of network structure (Borgatti et al., 2013). Examples of commonly examined workplace ties include communication, advice, support, friendship, and influence (Ibarra, 1993). Ties can be measured as simply existing or not, but are often measured in terms of strength, ranging from strong to weak (Granovetter, 1973). Strong ties tend to be long-standing relationships, characterized by affect and frequent contact. Strong ties carry with them a deeper sense of reciprocity, interest in the well-being of the other individual, and motivation to help. They often exist among members of cohesive groups in which interaction is common and shared norms guide behavior. Weak ties represent the opposite end of the spectrum — casual, distant, and superficial relationships.

The basic building blocks of networks are separate dyadic relationships (Brass & Krackhardt, 2012). In the example network (Fig. 1) there are eight individuals connected by twelve workplace relationships. Social network analysis extends beyond the study of singular relationships to examine the structure of interrelated dyads that constitute the network (Wasserman & Faust, 1994). Questions of interest include: how the dyads relate to each other, how the network structure affects different individuals in the network, and how individuals' characteristics as well as their ties influence outcomes. These analyses can allow for better informed decision-making, planning, and strategic action by bringing out information which would

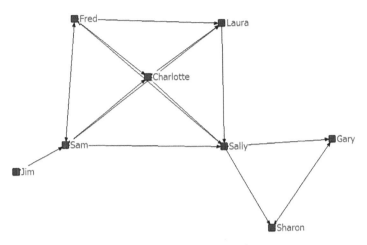

*Fig. 1.* Example Network.

normally seem invisible or attributable to different factors (Cross, Parker, Prusak, & Borgatti, 2001). In the remainder of this section, we provide a deeper discussion the connection between networks and individuals' well-being.

*Centrality*
Network centrality refers to the extent to which a person is connected to others in the network. In Fig. 1 Charlotte is the most central, whereas Jim is the most peripheral. The others fall somewhere along this spectrum. Given the historic focus in management research on networks such as advice, information sharing, and friendship, being central has generally been thought to be positive for individuals. Early observations comparing central individuals to those who were on the periphery found that isolation from the communication flow was associated with negative affect and diminished job satisfaction (cf. Roberts & O'Reilly, 1979). An abundance of evidence supports a positive connection between centrality and good performance (e.g., Cross & Cummings, 2004; Sparrowe, Liden, Wayne, & Kraimer, 2001) and job satisfaction (e.g., Ibarra & Andrews, 1993).

There are several reasons to assume that centrality (in workplace networks) is linked to employees' well-being. Central (rather than peripheral) individuals have a better vision of the network, so they do not waste time or endure stress by trying to figure out where to find resources (Krackhardt, 1990). Being central also conveys that the individual has power within the network (Brass, 1984, 1985; Brass & Burkhardt, 1993; Krackhardt, 1990), and thus individuals in those positions are often able to obtain better outcomes or receive better treatment (Brass & Krackhardt, 2012). Further, being a source of advice for people who themselves are highly central is positively associated with acceptance from peers (Ibarra & Andrews, 1993) and other forms of social support (Borgatti, Jones, & Everett, 1998).

However, more recent research suggests that there are potential downsides to centrality (Adler & Kwon, 2002). Central employees manage relationships with a large number of people and are disproportionally sought out for information and advice (Blau, 1964; Salancik & Pfeffer, 1974). Employees in central positions may become overwhelmed with information and requests from others and become overwhelmed by the effort required to maintain many relationships (Oldroyd & Morris, 2012; Soltis, Agneessens, Sasovova, & Labianca, 2013). Supporting this notion, Cullen, Gerbasi, and Chrobot-Mason (forthcoming) found that central individuals in workplace communication networks were more likely to experience role overload and ambiguity and ultimately lower levels of thriving. Star employees are especially likely to attract the attention of colleagues, placing them at risk of becoming overloaded (Oldroyd & Morris, 2012). Often attempts to enhance collaboration through new organizational structures or collaborative technologies actually intensify the collaborative demands on central, highly visible employees, instead of redistributing collaboration to underutilized employees (Cross & Gray, 2013).

### Structural Holes

Whereas centrality is primarily concerned with the size of the network (i.e., the number of connections an individual has), the structure of a person's network is also important to consider. Individuals who have relationships with people who are otherwise not connected are called brokers. They occupy a position in the network which provides advantages in information access, arbitrage or transfer, and translation (Burt, 1992). By connecting two otherwise unconnected people or groups, in other words, by "bridging a structural hole," the broker is in a unique position to access novel, nonredundant information (Burt, 1992). In this position, the broker can keep apart the two unconnected parties by playing the critical role of filtering and relaying information. The broker controls the flow of the information, placing this person in what is known as the *tertius gaudens* advantage (i.e., the third who benefits) in competitive or innovative situations.

Individuals in brokering positions also have the opportunity to bring people, groups, or parts of the network together to the benefit of all involved (*tertius iungens*) (Obstfeld, 2005). In organizations, this might mean connecting people with synergistic skills and knowledge or facilitating greater collaboration between different groups. Indeed, teams whose members have ties that span important organizational boundaries (e.g., function, geography, hierarchy) also have stronger performance (Reagans et al., 2004). Thus, brokers who act as "boundary spanners"[1] may gain favors or create obligations within their network that may benefit them in the long term (Brass & Krackhardt, 2012). They may also experience positive emotions from making connections that are beneficial to not only themselves but others as well.

Emerging research suggests that some individuals experience strain in brokering (Burt, Hogarth & Michaud, 2000; Xiao & Tsui, 2007) and boundary spanning positions (Kahn, Wolfe, Quinn, Snoek, & Rosenthal, 1964; Marrone, Tesluk, & Carson, 2007). To truly take advantage of structural holes, the individual must be integrated well enough into both groups to access potentially vital, novel information, as well as to be taken seriously when sharing information from another group. Developing relationships with this level of trust, in multiple social groups, requires considerable time investment, which may strain employees (Aldrich & Herker, 1977; Burt, 2015). Further, individuals engaged in boundary spanning activities often experience role overload as they try to manage their internal team responsibilities with their external activities (Kahn et al., 1964; Marrone et al., 2007), respond to different sets of expectations norms and demands from each group, as well as reconcile their own multiple identities that develop from participating in different groups (Hogg, Van Knippenberg, & Rast, 2012; Xiao & Tsui, 2007). Strain is especially likely when individuals act as intermediaries between people or groups in conflict (Aldrich & Herker, 1977; Burt, 2005).

*Embeddedness*
Other research suggests benefits related to being embedded in a group where there are strong relationships between most individuals. Research supporting this notion (e.g., Coleman, 1990; Granovetter, 2005) focused on the overall structure of the network, specifically the network's density. Network density refers to the number of relationships that exist within a network out of all the possible relationships that could exist (Wasserman & Faust, 1994). Groups with highly dense network structures are often described as high in social capital, which research has consistently been

found to be positively related to individual well-being and health (e.g., Helliwell & Putnam, 2004). Dense networks are notable for providing social support and safety to their members. Due to the high level of connectivity and strong ties, individuals embedded in dense networks tend to be aware of the needs and concerns of others in their network and quickly come to the support of other members (Adler & Kwon, 2002).

Dense networks also serve a role of propagating norms and expectations (Coleman, 1990) that can aid in creating more other-oriented behavior, civic behavior (Putnam, 1995) and even positive organizational citizenship behaviors (Lee, Mitchell, Sablynski, Burton, & Holtom, 2004). Within highly dense networks information travels quickly, thereby discouraging negative behaviors and generating trust because there is a risk to an individual's reputation (Brass, Butterfield, & Skaggs, 1998). Thus, in addition to providing a safe environment, in terms of support, closed networks also create a social environment where individuals become known for better or for worse. The term "embeddedness" is used to reflect the extent to which a "dyad's mutual contacts are connected to one another" (Granovetter, 1992, p. 35), and reflects the extent to which a person's actions are constrained by having many contacts who also know each other.

Building on the findings of early embeddedness research, researchers have recently become interested in the spread of gossip (both positive and negative) within networks as well as how gossip helps or hinders the individuals within the network (Burt & Knez, 1996; Ellwardt, Labianca, & Wittek, 2012). Positive gossip refers to being praised or defended by others and indicates that the members of the team support the target of the gossip (Ellwardt et al., 2012). Positive gossip serves to reinforce group norms and help maintain social control by praising those who exemplify the group ideals and helps create a sense of belongingness for the group members (Burt & Knez, 1996; Ellwardt et al., 2012). As such, Ellwardt and colleagues explain that positive gossip can boost one's reputation within the group, both when a person is the focus of the gossip as well as when one is spreading the positive gossip because these positions indicate that the actors are committed to the group norms. They explain that negative gossip also reinforces group norms, but rather than praising cooperating individuals, it sanctions those who violate group norms. For the person who is being gossiped about, negative gossip can hinder work-related success, reduce belonging, trust, and impede the building of network connections. Alternately, the person spreading negative gossip may benefit from transmitting this information as this act signals an understanding of group norms and a willingness to enforce them (Kniffin & Wilson, 2005).

Like centrality, sometimes an individual can be too embedded in their network. Oh et al. (2004) found that the benefits of embeddedness to a team's performance have a limit: some leads to good performance, but too much is stifling. Additionally, being excessively embedded in a network, without having diverse ties that reach outside of the closed network, can leave an actor with "redundant" information (Burt, 1992). Highly embedded networks can also constrain creativity and individuality because of a strong shared norms and expectations (Krackhardt, 1999). Some scholars have raised concerns that organizations attempts to develop closed; highly collaborative networks are merely ways to reinforce normative rules and ensure close monitoring and compliance (Barker, 1993). Given that well-being relies both on a sense of belonging as well as on autonomy (Ryan & Deci, 2000), embeddedness can both enable and hinder well-being.

*Negative Networks*
As mentioned previously, research examining networks and well-being has typically focused on networks that consist of either neutral, instrumental ties (e.g., advice or information ties) or positive affective ties (e.g., friendship, social support). However, a growing literature has examined the toll negative ties can take on employees. Although people usually report few ties such as incivility, negative gossip, or bullying, they attribute great importance to them (Casciaro & Lobo, 2008). Negative relationships are more potent than positive ones because of the increased cognitive functioning that negative ties create (Casciaro & Lobo, 2008; Labianca, Brass, & Gray, 1998; Parker et al., 2013). Negative ties tend to shift individuals' attention away from focusing on how to accomplish their task goals; employees spend cognitive resources analyzing their negative relationship and how best to navigate (often around) the person (Gerbasi, Porath, Parker, Cross, & Spreitzer, 2015; Parker et al., 2013). The distraction created by negative ties may explain why people who experience negative relationships do not learn and recall as well (Ellis, Moore, Varner, & Ottaway, 1997) and why negative ties weigh more heavily on outcomes, including harming job performance, promotions, and organizational attachment (Labianca & Brass, 2006). Negative ties between individuals in different teams also heighten the perception of conflict between the two teams — escalating the scope of the conflict; however, positive relationships do not have the same magnifying effect (Labianca et al., 1998). Parker et al. (2013) also found that employees who experienced the most negative interactions reported substantially less thriving.

The detrimental effects of negative ties are particularly salient in the workplace because task and work flow interdependence can make it difficult to severe negative ties (Labianca et al., 1998). For example, individuals are stuck with a negative relationship because of the reporting structure in an organization or because of membership on the same team. Further, the boarder network of relationships in which a person is embedded constrains how a person can handle the negative relationships they are involved in. Consider the example network in Fig. 1 and the following information: Fred and Sam are very close friends, Sally is Sam's wife, whom Fred has never gotten along with, and Fred thinks Sally is quite rude. For Fred to end the negative relationship with Sally, he would probably have to end his relationship with Sam which may be unlikely given their friendship. In sum, individuals' other network connections (often times positive ones) can constrain how they deal with negative ties. When interaction with a colleague is imposed for whatever reason, individuals may dread it, ruminate about future interactions, and feel their creativity or initiative is inhibited (Porath & Pearson, 2013).

Negative ties encourage people to separate from others in the workplace and reduce their sense of belonging (Dutton, 2003). Negative ties limit psychological safety (Edmondson, 1999), which may encourage individuals to retreat from others in their network, thus reducing the opportunity to learn (Casciaro & Lobo, 2008). Negative ties also represent blocked opportunities: information is more difficult to come by, resources are no longer accessed, and promotion opportunities are missed (Porath, Gerbasi, & Schorch, 2015).

# IMPLICATIONS FOR LEADERS

Given the importance of networks to leader and employee effectiveness as well as well-being, leaders need to understand their own social network and the network connecting their employees. Leaders in particular may find themselves in network positions that can have detrimental effects on their well-being (Balkundi & Kilduff, 2006; Daly & Finnigan, 2011). In addition to improving their own well-being, leaders can help employees develop networks that will promote (and not undermine) their well-being. There are many possibilities for leaders to improve their own well-being and to help promote the well-being of their employees.

*What Can Leaders Do to Improve Their Own Well-Being?*

Growing evidence suggests that central and brokering positions are important for leaders' own effectiveness and the performance of their teams (Balkundi & Harrison, 2006; Mehra et al., 2006). However, emerging research also suggests that there may be some perils associated with these "advantageous" positions. For example, being a source of information and expertise for colleagues makes a person valuable, but may result in overload if too many people depend on this single person. Leaders need to be particularly concerned as they tend to face more collaboration demands than other employees (Denison, Hooijberg, & Quinn, 1995). Thus, leaders need to take stock of their own network and identify if there are aspects of their network that may be undermining their well-being. Some individuals may be reluctant to intentionally shape their network because these activities seem insincere or self-serving (Casciaro, Gino, & Kouchaki, 2014). Leaders may feel better about taking steps to actively manage their network when they understand that these actions can provide benefit to others as well as themselves, including creating conditions that enhance everyone's well-being.

### Grow and Deepen Network Connections

If leaders are not well-connected, they are likely to experience a dearth of social support. Further, given the collaborative nature of their workplace, they may have difficulty finding meaning in their work and feeling energized by it. Leaders facing this issue need to take strategic steps to build their network. A common challenge for leaders is finding time to actively build their own network. For example, women leaders commonly reported that they could not possibly fit networking activities into their already busy schedule (Ely, Ibarra, & Kolb, 2011). Rethinking what constitutes networking and realizing that network building can be incorporated into daily work can help busy leaders overcome this barrier (Hewlett, Peraino, Sherbin, & Sumberg, 2010).

Individuals also have to be able and willing to leverage the relationships they have developed. Depending on the type of help or support that is needed, leaders need to ensure that they have built deep enough relationships and have diverse enough connections to provide the support they need. Building multiplex relationships is one useful way to maximize the benefits of each relationship and to optimize the number of relationships without losing resources (Oh et al., 2004). Multiplex ties help to create deeper relationships which can be leveraged and may mitigate the experience of overload from maintaining too many relationships.

*Minimize Collaboration Overload*

As mentioned previously, having more contacts is better, though only to a certain extent (Borgatti et al., 2013) – people cannot endlessly develop and manage relationships (Dunbar, 1992). Cross and Gray (2013) have found that many of the interactions that accumulate around leaders and place them in overloaded, "bottleneck" positions, are unnecessary or an unproductive use of time. They propose that leaders should start by identifying these "productivity-draining interactions" and find strategies to prevent becoming overloaded by their contacts. Leaders may re-direct unnecessary exchanges to someone better suited (either due to their role or skill set) to handle them (Goode, 1960). Among a number of others strategies (see Cross & Gray, 2013), this might also require re-allocating routine decisions, shifting part of the leader's role to others as a developmental opportunity, holding only necessary and efficient meetings, making information available through other people, websites, or mass communications, and creating buffers to limit the types of requests that reach the leader. Dean and Webb (2011) emphasize that leaders should focus on problems only they can address, let others know their priorities and filter information accordingly. Making these changes requires a concerted effort to reset workplace communication norms and culture (Dean & Webb, 2011), leaders should get assistance with this process if needed (e.g., coaching) to avoid falling into old traps (Cross & Gray, 2013).

*Manage the Tension of Being in the Middle*

Being in the middle (i.e., in boundary spanning or brokering positions) can be a difficult situation, requiring a lot of time and energy. This laborious work constitutes a large portion of the workload of higher-level mangers and leaders, because they often represent their groups to other parts of the organization as well as gather needed information and resources (Yip, Ernst, & Campbell, 2011). Further, leaders are often faced with the challenge of fostering greater levels of collaboration between groups with different interests and who may even be in conflict. To help groups move toward higher levels of intergroup collaboration, leaders must manage perceptions that they favor one group over the other (Hogg et al., 2012) and must help the groups avoid feelings of threat that can occur when disparate groups are asked to collaborate (Ernst & Chrobot-Mason, 2010). The leader's role is not to be a chameleon or to choose sides; instead, it is to facilitate a process by which group members can productively span boundaries. First, leaders help members of different groups understand their own strengths and needs as well as the strengths and needs of the other group. Then, they create opportunities for members of different groups to connect personally and discover similarities, shared values, and interests. These personal connections are an important means to overcome intergroup differences. As personal relationships form, a denser network is created between the groups helping to build mutual confidence and trust, which is the foundation for groups to build a shared direction and coordinate their efforts to achieve a common purpose (Chrobot-Mason, Cullen, & Altman, 2013). This approach can help relieve some of the identity-based tension that leaders feel and is also a means to over time shift boundary spanning responsibilities away from the leader to members of the group. When appropriate, leaders should encourage members of their own team to engage in boundary spanning to help offset the overload they may be experiencing.

## Improve Social Effectiveness

To access resources from their network individuals need to understand their colleagues and use that knowledge to influence them in ways that will provide the resources they desire (Wei, Chiang, & Wu, 2012). In other words they need political skill (Ferris et al., 2005) which consists of networking ability (i.e., ability to identify and develop diverse networks of relationships), social astuteness (i.e., ability to understand oneself, others, and their social interactions), apparent sincerity (i.e., ability to appear authentic, genuine, and honest to others), and interpersonal influence (i.e., ability to adjust behavior to elicit desired responses from others) (Ferris et al., 2007). Political skill helps individuals to deal more effectively with workplace stressors (e.g., Perrewé et al., 2004) by providing them with a greater sense of confidence and control and also likely providing them with greater access to information and resources in their work environment (Ferris et al., 2007). For example, recent research found that politically skilled individuals experience less role ambiguity when central to communication networks, suggesting that they are able to prioritize and strategically respond to information requests, while employees low in political skill may become confused about their role when communicating with many colleagues (Cullen et al., forthcoming). Leaders can enhance their political skill by receiving instruction and participating in experiential exercises, mentoring, coaching, feedback, case studies, and roleplaying, but political skill takes time to develop and is best gained through experience (Ferris, Perrewé, Anthony, & Gilmore, 2000; Perrewé, Ferris, Frink, & Anthony, 2000).

*Manage Negativity and Spark Energy in Your Relationships*
Negative interactions are unavoidable (Parker et al., 2013; Soltis et al., 2013), but there are ways to manage them that reduce their negative effect on well-being. First, and foremost, leaders are advised to try to minimize negative interactions where possible by working around or limiting contact with de-energizing individuals. Second, they should surround themselves with positive and energizing interactions, which can help act as a buffer to the negative interactions they do experience (Gerbasi et al., 2015; Parker et al., 2013). Third, leaders can bolster their well-being by focusing on creating energy in their relationships. To create energy in their interactions, leaders should foster conversations that explore possibilities and result in progress toward shared objectives (Cross, Baker, & Parker, 2003). This means looking for positive aspects of people's contributions and not shutting down ideas too early – instead identifying parts of the idea that help the work progress forward. Further, others feel energized when they believe the person they are connecting with is fully engaged in the conversation. To most effectively create energy in their interactions, leaders need to be mindful of their own energy levels, paying attention to how their energy levels shift throughout the day. With this knowledge, leaders can better structure their day and use relaxation and stress-reducing techniques to encourage more positive, effective, and energizing interactions with others (cf. Fritz, Lam, & Spreitzer, 2011).

## *What Can Leaders Do to Improve the Well-Being of Their Employees?*

As organizations increasingly rely on collaborative work, information overload has become a common experience for employees. Leaders can help to improve the well-being of their employees by looking for ways to minimize the overload many employees experience. The ease of capturing and analyzing the structure of social relationships has dramatically increased, offering new possibilities for leaders to manage the networks in their organization. Beyond investing in better understanding organizational networks through survey-based methodologies, many organizations are taking advantage of recent technological advances to collect data on interactions between employees (e.g., digital trace data, sociometric sensors; Kim, McFee, Olguin, Waber, & Pentland, 2012). Network analysis has traditionally been used to improve employee and organizational effectiveness and productivity; however, leaders can also use insights from these analyses to help improve the well-being of their employees.

*Redesign Jobs for Overloaded Employees*

Several scholars have highlighted the connection between job design, the networks employees accumulate, and their workplace experience (Grant, 2007; Grant & Parker, 2009). Beyond helping employees become aware of how their networks may be helping or hindering their well-being, leaders can take actions to alter employees' jobs to remove or minimize certain communication and collaboration interactions for overloaded employees. Leaders should prioritize helping overloaded employees because these employees are often stars in the organization (Oldroyd & Morris, 2012) and are at greater risk for leaving (Cross & Gray, 2013). Leaders may clarify expectations for information sharing, redefine the scope of employees' jobs, or have someone screen requests to reduce and prioritize interactions for overloaded employees. Further, leaders can identify other people who are on the periphery of the network, but have relevant knowledge and expertise and find ways to shift some collaborative connections to those individuals. This practice serves the dual purpose of relieving the overloaded employee and engaging the more isolated employee, which should improve everyone's well-being and productivity (for more suggestions see Cross & Gray, 2013).

*Establish Clear Collaboration Norms*

Although there has been a surge toward connectivity and collaboration in the workplace, it is important for leaders to critically assess where collaboration is and is not needed (Cross & Gray, 2013). This requires carefully deciding which groups and individuals need to be included on a project or in making a decision and setting workplace norms and expectations about when to consult with others and when to proceed independently. For example, W. L. Gore (Gore Creative Technologies Worldwide, 2015) has clear guidelines that associates have the freedom to make decisions that are above the "waterline," meaning that, if they put a "hole in the hull they will not sink the ship"; for any decisions below the waterline associates are expected to consult with others. For organizations with collaborative cultures like W. L. Gore to avoid the pitfalls of over collaborating, employees need simple, clear guidelines.

*Create a Workplace That Reinforces Well-Being*

In addition to helping employees better manage their work and collaboration load, changing the organizational culture can be an effective way of increasing well-being and reducing stress. Creating a culture which focuses on collective interest should promote giving behavior and meaningfulness

(Grant & Patil, 2012). Particularly if the organization is composed of a dense network, with strong ties between individuals, these positive norms will be reinforced (Coleman, 1990). Organizations that adapt this type of culture are thought to have a better chance of retaining their employees (Grant, 2012).

The existing social networks within organizations may be engaged to accelerate this process. Increasingly organizations are attempting to identify individuals in key (e.g., central and brokering) network positions and to work with them to influence their colleagues to adopt behaviors that will promote greater health and well-being and spread organizational norms that will reinforce these choices (Hollenbeck & Jamieson, 2015). These approaches have traditionally been used within companies to engage individuals in organizational changes and other strategic initiatives; however, research on community health and well-being initiatives suggests that these approaches could be successfully implemented in organization to help improve the health and well-being of individuals in their workplace (cf. Valente, 2010).

## Foster Energizing Relationships

Leaders can also promote productive, energizing relationships and minimize unproductive, de-energizing relationships in their groups. Research suggests that doing so, will improve job satisfaction (Venkataramani, Labianca, & Grosser, 2013) and more generally employees' well-being. For example, a network analysis of an oil and gas firm revealed that, despite a potentially mutually beneficial relationship between one unit in Africa and its sister unit in Europe, there was little exchange of ideas because the units were connected by a single, negative boundary spanning relationship (Parker et al., 2013). After learning this information, the manager took steps to promote greater interaction between others in the two units, eventually leading to more positive and beneficial relationships. Research by Edward Lawler and his colleagues (Lawler & Yoon, 1993, 1996) shows that repeated interactions that have mutually rewarding positive outcomes tend to produce energizing relationships. Projects and workflows which create consistent task interdependence (as opposed to frequently switching team members) should allow for energizing relationships to grow and flourish. Creating a culture of open communication can foster trust and relationship building that will serve to create energy and promote well-being.

The formal structure of an organization and job design can create interactions that would normally not persist due to personal differences, disagreements, and negative emotion (Labianca & Brass, 2006). Individuals with many negative ties are less satisfied with their work and being disliked by several coworkers has reputation effects that can hinder the individual's position in the organization. When negative ties are unable to be mediated or resolved, there are several possible paths of actions. Leaders can make changes to the workflow so that the people involved in the negative ties do not have to interact with one another (Parker et al., 2013). They should also help employees with negative relationships develop valued, positive relationships to keep the employee from being relegated to the periphery of the networks. The key is to help employees see negative ties as an opportunity for personal development because these ties may provide feedback regarding how they are viewed by others (Labianca & Brass, 2006).

# DIRECTIONS FOR FUTURE RESEARCH

The management field has witnessed an explosion of research on networks (Brass & Krackhardt, 2012). The majority of this research has focused on how networks are important for obtaining instrumental benefits. Growing research is acknowledging the importance of networks for employee well-being and there are several existing areas in need of further research.

*Positive versus Negative Ties*

Growing research suggests that incivility in the workplace is a major issue impacting the well-being of employees. In 1998, 25% of employees reported being treated rudely at work at least once a week, that percentage rose to over 50% in 2011 (Porath & Pearson, 2013). Recent research also shows the benefits of civility in terms of leadership, competence, and performance (Porath et al., 2015), but little is known about how civility and incivility actually spread through networks and how different working conditions facilitate and/or hinder the spread of workplace civility. Further, research is needed to determine how to promote civility and minimize incivility in the workplace. Recent research by O'Connor and Cavanagh (2013) found that individuals who received coaching reported greater well-being as well as improved communication exchanges, this improvement in well-being spread to people around the coached employee. This research suggests that the benefits of coaching could spread to others in the workplace, perhaps creating an expanding network of civil interactions.

Most of the current research on social networks focuses on positive or negative ties exclusively, but to gain a full picture of the support and strain an individual faces positive and negative ties need to be considered at the same time. These ties do not always operate separately or in opposite directions, but might work in combination (Venkataramani et al., 2013). For example, what is the implication of having a negative tie to someone who has many positives ties? Does this type of network lead to isolation and alienation? Alternatively, does having a negative tie to someone who has many other negative ties create a bonding experience for individuals (i.e., create a commonality that was not otherwise there)?

There are also questions regarding whether positivity and negativity spread through the network in the same way. Some initial evidence (Ellwardt et al., 2012) suggests they take different paths. Whereas positive interactions appear to be able to spread through networks, negative interactions tend to be centralized around certain individuals. This suggests that negativity could be contained and managed, but more research is needed to understand the mechanisms by which positive and negative ties spread through networks.

### Managing the Boundary Spanning Role

As we have described, substantial research has demonstrated the instrumental advantages of occupying brokering and boundary spanning positions. Growing research suggests that these positions can cause individuals to experience strain which can negatively impact well-being. Brokering positions are assertive and agentic by nature (Brands & Kilduff, 2013) and can benefit individuals especially when they are perceived as acting with warmth and compassion (Casciaro & Lobo, 2008). However, this may be a difficult perception to achieve when actively managing the interactions between people or groups who are not connected. Research is needed to understand how individuals build relationships with the required trust to access information and collaborate effectively without embedding themselves excessively in a network (i.e., while maintaining their broker position). Indeed, creating trusting relationships and avoiding being seen as an outsider or opportunist is a major challenge for leaders who are trying to reach into other groups. Further, brokers' ties are likely to decay more rapidly than the ties of individuals who are embedded in dense networks (Burt, 2010). It is unclear what effect this churning of networking ties has on brokers' well-being, but it reasonable to assume that it could be detrimental as they maintain fewer long-term relationships.

## Personality and Social Competencies

Network researchers have begun to examine how the personalities of individuals within the network influence their patterns of interacting and the effects they have on others. The majority of research has focused on whether certain personality traits (e.g., self-monitoring, the Big Five) are predictive of centrality and brokering positions (cf. Fang, Landis, Zhang, Anderson, & Shaw, Kilduff, 2015). However, research is needed to understand whether individuals with certain characteristics such as conscientiousness, who are sought for advice may also be most at risk of becoming overloaded in the network, and may be the individuals least able to say no to excessive demands. Further research is also needed to examine how personality predicts individuals' network position in specific contexts and with regard to specific types of networks. For example, recent research found that extroverts energize their teammates when there is agreement on the path forward, but when task conflict exists, extraverts do not have the same energizing effects (Cullen, Leroy, & Gerbasi, 2015).

Additional research is needed to understand how not only personality, but also how individuals' social competencies influence the relationship between their network position and their well-being. Cullen et al. (forthcoming) provided initial evidence that political skill can help employees deal more effectively with some demands of central positions (i.e., role ambiguity), but found that political skill did not influence their experience of role overload. Future research may consider which personal characteristics could help employees to experience less overload from many network connections. Research is also needed to identify the traits and competencies that could help people to manage the demands of brokering/boundary spanning positions. Political skill may help individual's manage the strain associated with being in the middle of different groups as these individuals are thought to develop friendships easily and build beneficial coalitions and alliances (Ferris et al., 2007). A recent review by Munyon, Summers, Thompson, and Ferris (2015) found very few studies examining political skill and networking or network position. Gaining a better understanding the connection between political skill, the network's employees develop, and their experience as a result of their network connections is an important area for future research. This general line of research could help organizations select people who could sustain themselves in central and brokering positions.

## *Context*

Due to the nature of network studies (generally in-depth analysis of one organizational setting), little is known about how context affects the creation of positive and negative resources that are conveyed through networks. It has been argued the context of work can influence the creation of energy in the workplace by influencing the patterns and types of interactions individuals have during their work day (Quinn & Dutton, 2005; Quinn et al., 2012), but there has been very little comparative research examining the types of affective ties fostered by different types of work environments. Researchers may examine how organizational change influences the creation of positive and negative resources within networks (Jansen, 2004). This focus is particularly relevant as positive relationships, particularly energizing relationships, motivate individuals. If employees are positively inclined and energized, it may improve the success of the organizational change initiative. Further, contextual factors may determine whether certain network positions are beneficial or detrimental to an individual's well-being.

## CONCLUSION

Scholars have long highlighted the importance of relationship for individuals' well-being. In the workplace, relationships are only likely to become more important for understanding employees' work experience as organizations increasingly engage in interdependent, knowledge-based work. Social network concepts and methods have the promise to offer new insights into employee well-being. These insights are of critical importance to leaders as they are responsible for maintaining not only their own well-being, but also the well-being of their employees. In this chapter we describe emerging research demonstrating the connection between networks and well-being. In doing so, we hope to encourage an increased focus among management scholars in understanding not only the instrumental outcomes of networks, but also how workplace networks affect affective outcomes, most notably employee well-being.

# NOTE

1. It should be noted that brokers are not necessarily boundary spanners as they could occupy structural holes within the same group and boundary spanners are not necessarily brokers as other people in their group could have ties to the other group as well. However, commonly brokers do span boundaries as their ties reach into different clusters within the network that consist of different organizational groups.

# REFERENCES

Adler, P. S., & Kwon, S. W. (2002). Social capital: Prospects for a new concept. *Academy of Management Review*, 27(1), 17–40.

Aldrich, H., & Herker, D. (1977). Boundary spanning roles and organizational structure. *Academy of Management Journal*, 2(2), 217–230.

Baker, W., Cross, R., & Wooten, M. (2003). Positive organizational network analysis and energizing relationships. In K. S. Cameron, J. E. Dutton, & R. E. Quinn (Eds.), *Positive organizational scholarship: Foundations of a new discipline* (pp. 328–342). San Francisco, CA: Berrett-Koehler Publishers.

Balkundi, P., & Harrison, D. A. (2006). Ties, leaders, and time in teams: Strong inference about network structure's effects on team viability and performance. *Academy of Management Journal*, 49(1), 49–68.

Balkundi, P., & Kilduff, M. (2006). The ties that lead: A social network approach to leadership. *The Leadership Quarterly*, 17(4), 419–439.

Barker, J. R. (1993). Tightening the iron cage: Concertive control in self-managing teams. *Administrative Science Quarterly*, 38(3), 408–437.

Barsade, S. G. (2002). The ripple effect: Emotional contagion and its influence on group behavior. *Administrative Science Quarterly*, 47(4), 644–675.

Blau, P. M. (1964). *Exchange and power in everyday life*. New York, NY: Wiley.

Borgatti, S. P., & Cross, R. (2003). A relational view of information seeking and learning in social networks. *Management Science*, 49(4), 432–445.

Borgatti, S. P., Everett, M. G., & Johnson, J. C. (2013). *Analyzing social networks*. Los Angeles, CA: Sage Publications Limited.

Borgatti, S. P., Jones, C., & Everett, M. G. (1998). Network measures of social capital. *Connections*, 21(2), 27–36.

Brands, R. A., & Kilduff, M. (2013). Just like a woman? Effects of gender-biased perceptions of friendship network brokerage on attributions and performance. *Organization Science*, 25(5), 1530–1548.

Brass, D. J. (1984). Being in the right place: A structural analysis of individual influence in an organization. *Administrative Science Quarterly*, 29(4), 518–539.

Brass, D. J. (1985). Men's and women's networks: A study of interaction patterns and influence in an organization. *Academy of Management Journal*, 28(2), 327–343.

Brass, D. J., & Burkhardt, M. E. (1993). Potential power and power use: An investigation of structure and behavior. *Academy of Management Journal*, 36(3), 441–470.

Brass, D. J., Butterfield, K. D., & Skaggs, B. C. (1998). Relationships and unethical behavior: A social network perspective. *Academy of Management Review, 23*(1), 14–31.

Brass, D. J., Galaskiewicz, J., Greve, H. R., & Tsai, W. (2004). Taking stock of networks and organizations: A multilevel perspective. *Academy of Management Journal, 47*(6), 795–817.

Brass, D. J., & Krackhardt, D. M. (2012). Power, politics, and social networks in organizations. In G. R. Ferris & D. C. Treadway (Eds.), *Politics in organizations: Theory and research considerations* (pp. 355–375). New York, NY: Routledge.

Burt, R. S. (1992). *Structural holes*. Cambridge, MA: Harvard University Press.

Burt, R. S. (2005). *Brokerage and closure: An introduction to social capital*. Oxford: Oxford University Press.

Burt, R. S. (2010). *Neighbor networks*. Oxford, UK: Oxford University Press.

Burt, R. S. (2015). Reinforced structural holes. *Social Networks, 43*, 149–161.

Burt, R. S., Hogarth, R. M., & Michaud, C. (2000). The social capital of French and American managers. *Organization Science, 11*(2), 123–147.

Burt, R. S., & Knez, M. (1996). Trust and third-party gossip. In R. M. Kramer & T. R. Tyler (Eds.), *Trust in organizations: Frontiers of theory and research* (pp. 68–89). Thousand Oaks, CA: Sage.

Butts, M. M., Becker, W. J., & Boswell, W. R. (2015). Hot buttons and time sinks: The effects of electronic communication during nonwork time on emotions and work-nonwork conflict. *Academy of Management Journal, 58*(3), 763–788.

Carter, D. R., DeChurch, L. A., Braun, M. T., & Contractor, N. S. (2015). Social network approaches to leadership: An integrative conceptual review. *Journal of Applied Psychology, 100*(3), 597–622.

Casciaro, T., Gino, F., & Kouchaki, M. (2014). The contaminating effects of building instrumental ties how networking can make us feel dirty. *Administrative Science Quarterly, 59*(4), 705–735.

Casciaro, T., & Lobo, M. S. (2008). When competence is irrelevant: The role of interpersonal affect in task-related ties. *Administrative Science Quarterly, 53*(4), 655–684.

Chrobot-Mason, D., Cullen, K., & Altman, D. (2013). Leveraging networks through boundary spanning leadership. In J. Nickerson & R. Sanders (Eds.), *Tackling wicked government problems* (pp. 101–118). Arlington, VA: Oakland Street Publishing.

Clifton, D. O., & Harter, J. K. (2003). Investing in strengths. In K. S. Cameron, J. E. Dutton, & R. E. Quinn (Eds.), *Positive organizational scholarship: Foundations of a new discipline* (pp. 111–121). San Francisco, CA: Berrett-Koehler Publishers.

Coleman, J. S. (1990). *Equality and achievement in education*. Boulder, CO: Westview Press.

Cross, R., Baker, W., & Parker, A. (2003). What creates energy in organizations? *MIT Sloan Management Review, 44*(4), 51–56.

Cross, R., & Cummings, J. N. (2004). Tie and network correlates of individual performance in knowledge-intensive work. *Academy of Management Journal, 47*(6), 928–937.

Cross, R., & Gray, P. (2013). Where has the time gone? Addressing collaboration overload in a networked economy. *California Management Review, 56*(1), 50–66.

Cross, R., Parker, A., Prusak, L., & Borgatti, S. P. (2001). Knowing what we know: Supporting knowledge creation and sharing in social networks. *Organizational Dynamics, 30*(2), 100–120.

Cullen, K., Gerbasi, A., & Chrobot-Mason, D. (forthcoming). Thriving in central network positions: The role of political skill. *Journal of Management*.

Cullen, K., Leroy, H., & Gerbasi, A., (2015). Unraveling ties that link extraversion and proactive performance in teams. Paper presented at the Society for Industrial and Organizational Psychology, 30th Annual Meeting, Philadelphia, PA.

Daly, A. J., & Finnigan, K. S. (2011). The ebb and flow of social network ties between district leaders under high-stakes accountability. *American Educational Research Journal*, *48*(1), 39–79.

Dean, D., & Webb, C. (2011). Recovering from information overload. *McKinsey Quarterly*, *1*, 80–88.

Denison, D. R., Hooijberg, R., & Quinn, R. E. (1995). Paradox and performance: Toward a theory of behavioral complexity in managerial leadership. *Organization Science*, *6*(5), 524–540.

Diener, E. (2000). Subjective well-being: The science of happiness and a proposal for a national index. *American Psychologist*, *55*(1), 34–43.

Diener, E., Ng, W., Harter, J., & Arora, R. (2010). Wealth and happiness across the world: Material prosperity predicts life evaluation, whereas psychosocial prosperity predicts positive feeling. *Journal of Personality and Social Psychology*, *99*(1), 52.

Diener, E., Suh, E. M., Lucas, R. E., & Smith, H. L. (1999). Subjective well-being: Three decades of progress. *Psychological Bulletin*, *125*(2), 276–302.

Diener, E., Tay, L., & Meyers, D. G. (2011). The religion paradox: If religion makes people happy, why are so many dropping out? *Journal of Personality and Social Psychology*, *101*(6), 1278–1290.

Dunbar, R. I. (1992). Time: A hidden constraint on the behavioural ecology of baboons. *Behavioral Ecology and Sociobiology*, *31*(1), 35–49.

Dunn, E. W., Aknin, L. B., & Norton, M. I. (2008). Spending money on others promotes happiness. *Science*, *319*(5870), 1687–1688.

Dutton, J. E. (2003). *Energize your workplace: How to create and sustain high-quality connections at work*. San Francisco, CA: Jossey-Bass.

Dutton, J. E., & Heaphy, E. D. (2003). The power of high-quality connections. *Positive organizational scholarship: Foundations of a new discipline*, *3*, 263–278.

Edmondson, A. (1999). Psychological safety and learning behavior in work teams. *Administrative Science Quarterly*, *44*(2), 350–383.

Eisenberger, R., Stinglhamber, F., Vandenberghe, C., Sucharski, I. L., & Rhoades, L. (2002). Perceived supervisor support: Contributions to perceived organizational support and employee retention. *Journal of Applied Psychology*, *87*(3), 565–573.

Ellis, H. C., Moore, B. A., Varner, L. J., & Ottaway, S. A. (1997). Depressed mood, task organization, cognitive interference, and memory: Irrelevant thoughts predict recall performance. *Journal of Social Behavior & Personality*, *12*(2), 453–470.

Ellwardt, L., Labianca, G. J., & Wittek, R. (2012). Who are the objects of positive and negative gossip at work? A social network perspective on workplace gossip. *Social Networks*, *34*(2), 193–205.

Ely, R. J., Ibarra, H., & Kolb, D. M. (2011). Taking gender into account: Theory and design for women's leadership development programs. *Academy of Management Learning & Education*, *10*(3), 474–493.

Ernst, C., & Chrobot-Mason, D. (2010). *Boundary spanning leadership: Six practices for solving problems, driving innovation, and transforming organizations*. New York, NY: McGraw Hill Professional.

Fang, R., Landis, B., Zhang, Z., Anderson, M. H., Shaw, J. D., & Kilduff, M. (2015). Integrating personality and social networks: A meta-analysis of personality, network position, and work outcomes in organizations. *Organization Science, 26*(4), 1243–1260.

Ferris, G. R., Perrewé, P. L., Anthony, W. P., & Gilmore, D. C. (2000). Political skill at work. *Organizational Dynamics, 28*(4), 25–37.

Ferris, G. R., Treadway, D. C., Kolodinsky, R. W., Hochwarter, W. A., Kacmar, C. J., Douglas, C., & Frink, D. D. (2005). Development and validation of the political skill inventory. *Journal of Management, 31*(1), 126–152.

Ferris, G. R., Treadway, D. C., Perrewé, P. L., Brouer, R. L., Douglas, C., & Lux, S. (2007). Political skill in organizations. *Journal of Management, 33*(3), 290–320.

Fowler, J. H., & Christakis, N. A. (2008). Dynamic spread of happiness in a large social network: Longitudinal analysis over 20 years in the Framingham heart study. *British Medical Journal, 337*, a2338.

Fritz, C., Lam, C. F., & Spreitzer, G. M. (2011). It's the little things that matter: An examination of knowledge workers' energy management. *The Academy of Management Perspectives, 25*(3), 28–39.

Gerbasi, A., Porath, C. L., Parker, A., Cross, R., & Spreitzer, G. (2015). Destructive de-energizing relationships: How thriving buffers their effect on performance. *Journal of Applied Psychology, 100*(5), 1423–1433.

Global Human Capital Trends. (2014). *Engaging the 21st-century workforce.* Report. Deloitte Consulting LLP and Bersin. Retrieved from https://www2.deloitte.com/content/dam/Deloitte/ar/Documents/human-capital/arg_hc_global-human-capital-trends-2014_0906 2014%20(1).pdf

Goode, W. J. (1960). A theory of role strain. *American Sociological Review, 25*(4), 483–496.

Gore Creative Technologies Worldwide. (2015). *What we believe.* Retrieved from http://www.gore.com/en_xx/careers/whoweare/whatwebelieve/gore-culture.html

Granovetter, M. S. (1973). The strength of weak ties. *American Journal of Sociology, 78*(6), 1360–1380.

Granovetter, M. S. (1992). Economic institutions as social constructions: A framework for analysis. *Acta Sociologica, 35*(1), 3–11.

Granovetter, M. S. (2005). The impact of social structure on economic outcomes. *Journal of Economic Perspectives, 19*(1), 33–50.

Grant, A. M. (2007). Relational job design and the motivation to make a prosocial difference. *Academy of Management Review, 32*(2), 393–417.

Grant, A. M. (2012). Giving time, time after time: Work design and sustained employee participation in corporate volunteering. *Academy of Management Review, 37*(4), 589–615.

Grant, A. M., & Dutton, J. (2012). Beneficiary or benefactor are people more prosocial when they reflect on receiving or giving? *Psychological Science, 23*(9), 1033–1039.

Grant, A. M., & Parker, S. K. (2009). 7 redesigning work design theories: The rise of relational and proactive perspectives. *The Academy of Management Annals, 3*(1), 317–375.

Grant, A. M., & Patil, S. V. (2012). Challenging the norm of self-interest: Minority influence and transitions to helping norms in work units. *Academy of Management Review, 37*(4), 547–568.

Griffin, M. A., Neal, A., & Parker, S. K. (2007). A new model of work role performance: Positive behavior in uncertain and interdependent contexts. *Academy of Management Journal, 50*(2), 327–347.

Heaney, C. A., & Israel, B. A. (2008). Social networks and social support. *Health Behavior and Health Education: Theory, Research, and Practice, 4*, 189–210.

Helliwell, J. F., & Putnam, R. D. (2004). The social context of well-being. *Philosophical Transactions-Royal Society of London Series B Biological Sciences, 359*(1449), 1435–1446.

Hewlett, S. A., Peraino, K., Sherbin, L., & Sumberg, K. (2010). *The sponsor effect: Breaking through the last glass ceiling*. Cambridge, MA: Harvard University Press.

Hogg, M. A., Van Knippenberg, D., & Rast, D. E. (2012). Intergroup leadership in organizations: Leading across group and organizational boundaries. *Academy of Management Review, 37*(2), 232–255.

Hollenbeck, J. R., & Jamieson, B. B. (2015). Human capital, social capital, and social network analysis: Implications for strategic human resource management. *The Academy of Management Perspectives, 29*(3), 370–385.

Humphrey, S. E., Nahrgang, J. D., & Morgeson, F. P. (2007). Integrating motivational, social, and contextual work design features: A meta-analytic summary and theoretical extension of the work design literature. *Journal of Applied Psychology, 92*(5), 1332–1356.

Ibarra, H. (1993). Personal networks of women and minorities in management: A conceptual framework. *Academy of Management Review, 18*(1), 56–87.

Ibarra, H., & Andrews, S. B. (1993). Power, social influence, and sense making: Effects of network centrality and proximity on employee perceptions. *Administrative Science Quarterly, 38*(2), 277–303.

Ilgen, D. R., Hollenbeck, J. R., Johnson, M., & Jundt, D. (2005). Teams in organizations: From input-process-output models to IMOI models. *Annual Review of Psychology, 56*, 517–543.

Jansen, K. (2004). From persistence to pursuit: A longitudinal examination of momentum during the early stages of strategic change. *Organization Science, 15*, 276–294.

Kahn, R. L., Wolfe, D. M., Quinn, R. P., Snoek, J. D., & Rosenthal, R. A. (1964). *Organizational stress: Studies in role conflict and ambiguity*. New York, NY: Wiley.

Kawachi, I., & Berkman, L. F. (2001). Social ties and mental health. *Journal of Urban Health, 78*(3), 458–467.

Kim, T., McFee, E., Olguin, D. O., Waber, B., & Pentland, A. (2012). Sociometric badges: Using sensor technology to capture new forms of collaboration. *Journal of Organizational Behavior, 33*(3), 412–427.

Kniffin, K. M., & Wilson, D. S. (2005). Utilities of gossip across organizational levels: Multilevel selection, free-riders, and teams. *Human Nature, 16*(3), 278–292.

Krackhardt, D. (1990). Assessing the political landscape: Structure, cognition, and power in organizations. *Administrative Science Quarterly, 35*(2), 342–369.

Krackhardt, D. (1999). The ties that torture: Simmelian tie analysis in organizations. *Research in the Sociology of Organizations, 16*(1), 183–210.

Labianca, G., & Brass, D. J. (2006). Exploring the social ledger: Negative relationships and negative asymmetry in social networks in organizations. *Academy of Management Review, 31*(3), 596–614.

Labianca, G., Brass, D. J., & Gray, B. (1998). Social networks and perceptions of intergroup conflict: The role of negative relationships and third parties. *Academy of Management Journal, 41*(1), 55–67.

Lawler, E. J., & Yoon, J. (1993). Power and the emergence of commitment behavior in negotiated exchange. *American Sociological Review, 58*(4), 465–481.

Lawler, E. J., & Yoon, J. (1996). Commitment in exchange relations: Test of a theory of relational cohesion. *American Sociological Review, 61*(1), 89–108.

Lee, T. W., Mitchell, T. R., Sablynski, C. J., Burton, J. P., & Holtom, B. C. (2004). The effects of job embeddedness on organizational citizenship, job performance, volitional absences, and voluntary turnover. *Academy of Management Journal, 47*(5), 711–722.

Marrone, J. A., Tesluk, P. E., & Carson, J. B. (2007). A multilevel investigation of antecedents and consequences of team member boundary-spanning behavior. *Academy of Management Journal, 50*(6), 1423–1439.

Mehra, A., Dixon, A. L., Brass, D. J., & Robertson, B. (2006). The social network ties of group leaders: Implications for group performance and leader reputation. *Organization Science, 17*(1), 64–79.

Mogilner, C., Chance, Z., & Norton, M. I. (2012). Giving time gives you time. *Psychological Science, 23*(10), 1233–1238.

Munyon, T. P., Summers, J. K., Thompson, K. M., & Ferris, G. R. (2015). Political skill and work outcomes: A theoretical extension, meta-analytic investigation, and agenda for the future. *Personnel Psychology, 68*(1), 143–184.

Myers, D. G. (2000). The funds, friends, and faith of happy people. *American Psychologist, 55*(1), 56–67.

Obstfeld, D. (2005). Social networks, the tertius iungens orientation, and involvement in innovation. *Administrative Science Quarterly, 50*(1), 100–130.

O'Connor, S., & Cavanagh, M. (2013). The coaching ripple effect: The effects of developmental coaching on wellbeing across organisational networks. *Psychology of Well-Being, 3*(1), 1–23.

Oh, H., Chung, M. H., & Labianca, G. (2004). Group social capital and group effectiveness: The role of informal socializing ties. *Academy of Management Journal, 47*(6), 860–875.

Oldroyd, J. B., & Morris, S. S. (2012). Catching falling stars: A human resource response to social capital's detrimental effect of information overload on star employees. *Academy of Management Review, 37*(3), 396–418.

Parker, A., Gerbasi, A., & Porath, C. L. (2013). The effects of de-energizing ties in organizations and how to manage them. *Organizational Dynamics, 42*(2), 110–118.

Perrewé, P. L., Ferris, G. R., Frink, D. D., & Anthony, W. P. (2000). Political skill: An antidote for workplace stressors. *The Academy of Management Executive, 14*(3), 115–123.

Perrewé, P. L., Zellars, K. L., Ferris, G. R., Rossi, A. M., Kacmar, C. J., & Ralston, D. A. (2004). Neutralizing job stressors: Political skill as an antidote to the dysfunctional consequences of role conflict. *Academy of Management Journal, 47*(1), 141–152.

Porath, C. L., Gerbasi, A., & Schorch, S. L. (2015). Effects of civility on advice, leadership, and performance. *Journal of Applied Psychology, 100*(5), 1527–1541.

Porath, C. L., & Pearson, C. (2013). The price of incivility. *Harvard Business Review, 91*(1–2), 115–121.

Porath, C. L., Spreitzer, G., Gibson, C., & Garnett, F. G. (2012). Thriving at work: Toward its measurement, construct validation, and theoretical refinement. *Journal of Organizational Behavior, 33*(2), 250–275.

Putnam, R. D. (1995). Bowling alone: America's declining social capital. *Journal of Democracy, 6*(1), 65–78.

Quinn, R. W., & Dutton, J. E. (2005). Coordination as energy-in-conversation. *Academy of Management Review, 30*(1), 36–57.

Quinn, R. W., Spreitzer, G. M., & Lam, C. F. (2012). Building a sustainable model of human energy in organizations: Exploring the critical role of resources. *The Academy of Management Annals, 6*(1), 337–396.

Reagans, R., Zuckerman, E., & McEvily, B. (2004). How to make the team: Social networks vs. demography as criteria for designing effective teams. *Administrative Science Quarterly, 49*(1), 101–133.

Roberts, K. H., & O'Reilly, C. A. (1979). Some correlations of communication roles in organizations. *Academy of Management Journal, 22*(1), 42−57.

Rosso, B. D., Dekas, K. H., & Wrzesniewski, A. (2010). On the meaning of work: A theoretical Integration and review. *Research in Organizational Behavior, 30*, 91−127.

Ryan, R. M., & Deci, E. L. (2000). Self-determination theory and the facilitation of intrinsic motivation, social development, and well-being. *American Psychologist, 55*, 68−78.

Salancik, G. R., & Pfeffer, J. (1974). The bases and use of power in organizational decision making: The case of a university. *Administrative Science Quarterly, 19*(4), 453−473.

Sauter, S. L., Murphy, L. R., & Hurrell, J. J. (1990). Prevention of work-related psychological disorders: A national strategy proposed by the National Institute for Occupational Safety and Health (NIOSH). *American Psychologist, 45*, 1146−1158.

Soltis, S. M., Agneessens, F., Sasovova, Z., & Labianca, G. J. (2013). A social network perspective on turnover intentions: The role of distributive justice and social support. *Human Resource Management, 52*(4), 561−584.

Sparrowe, R. T., Liden, R. C., Wayne, S. J., & Kraimer, M. L. (2001). Social networks and the performance of individuals and groups. *Academy of Management Journal, 44*(2), 316−325.

Spreitzer, G., Porath, C. L., & Gibson, C. B. (2012). Toward human sustainability: How to enable more thriving at work. *Organizational Dynamics, 41*(2), 155−162.

Spreitzer, G. M., Sutcliffe, K., Dutton, J., Sonenshein, S., & Grant, A. M. (2005). A socially embedded model of thriving at work. *Organization Science, 16*(5), 537−549.

Stevenrink, N., & Lindenberg, S. (2006). Which social needs are important for subjective well-being? What happens to them with aging? *Psychology and Aging, 21*(2), 281−290.

Strikwerda, J., & Stoelhorst, J. W. (2009). The emergence and evolution of the multidimensional organization. *California Management Review, 51*(4), 11−31.

Tay, L., & Diener, E. (2011). Needs and subjective well-being around the world. *Journal of Personality and Social Psychology, 101*(2), 354.

Taylor, J., & Turner, R. J. (2001). A longitudinal study of the role and significance of mattering to others for depressive symptoms. *Journal of Health and Social Behavior, 42*(3), 310−325.

Totterdell, P., Wall, T., Holman, D., Diamond, H., & Epitropaki, O. (2004). Affect networks: A structural analysis of the relationship between work ties and job-related affect. *Journal of Applied Psychology, 89*(5), 854−867.

Valente, T. W. (2010). *Social networks and health: Models, methods, and applications.* New York, NY: Oxford University Press.

Venkataramani, V., Labianca, G. J., & Grosser, T. (2013). Positive and negative workplace relationships, social satisfaction, and organizational attachment. *Journal of Applied Psychology, 98*(6), 1028−1039.

Wasserman, S., & Faust, K. (1994). *Social network analysis: Methods and applications.* New York, NY: Cambridge University Press.

Wei, L. Q., Chiang, F. F., & Wu, L. Z. (2012). Developing and utilizing network resources: Roles of political skill. *Journal of Management Studies, 49*(2), 381−402.

Xiao, Z., & Tsui, A. S. (2007). When brokers may not work: The cultural contingency of social capital in Chinese high-tech firms. *Administrative Science Quarterly, 52*(1), 1−31.

Yip, J., Ernst, C., & Campbell, M. (2011). *Boundary spanning leadership.* Greensboro, NC: Center for Creative Leadership.

# DO YOU BELIEVE WHAT I BELIEVE? A THEORETICAL MODEL OF CONGRUENCE IN FOLLOWER ROLE ORIENTATION AND ITS EFFECTS ON MANAGER AND SUBORDINATE OUTCOMES

Melissa K. Carsten, Mary Uhl-Bien and
Tracy L. Griggs

## ABSTRACT

*Building upon relational leadership theory, we develop a theoretical model examining the association between leader-follower congruence in follower role orientation and manager and subordinate relational and well-being outcomes. Follower role orientation represents individuals' beliefs regarding the best way to enact a follower role. We predict that managers and subordinates who share similar role orientations will experience higher quality leader-member exchange (LMX) relationships and greater eustress than those who differ in their follower role orientations. Propositions are presented for direct effects between congruence and stress and indirect*

The Role of Leadership in Occupational Stress
Research in Occupational Stress and Well Being, Volume 14, 91–114
Copyright © 2016 by Emerald Group Publishing Limited
All rights of reproduction in any form reserved
ISSN: 1479-3555/doi:10.1108/S1479-355520160000014004

*effects through LMX. Our theoretical model contributes to nascent research on followership by offering greater understanding of manager and subordinate beliefs regarding how followers should enact their roles, and the importance of considering leader (i.e., manager) as well as follower outcomes in the workplace. It also extends current thinking about stress as an important outcome of leader-follower relationships.*

**Keywords:** Followership; leadership; role orientations; congruence analysis; eustress; distress

The leadership literature has documented the many important traits and characteristics that leaders bring to the leadership relationship (Yukl, 2012). Yet, fewer studies have examined the unique characteristics of followers and how these characteristics impact leader-follower interactions (Baker, 2007; Bligh, 2011; Collinson, 2006; Crossman & Crossman, 2011; Lapierre & Carsten, 2014). In emerging research on followership, scholars are beginning to explore follower traits and characteristics to understand their impact on leaders and the leadership process (Carsten, Uhl-Bien, West, Patera, & McGregor, 2010; Howell & Mendez, 2008; Uhl-Bien, Riggio, Lowe, & Carsten, 2014). One stream of research in this area is follower role orientation theory (Carsten, Uhl-Bien, & Jayawickrema, 2013; Uhl-Bien et al., 2014). Follower role orientation theory describes the beliefs that individuals hold regarding the best way to enact a follower role and the relationship between these beliefs and followership outcomes (Carsten et al., 2013). It examines role orientations not as overt behaviors, but as "trait-like" belief systems regarding the follower role in organizations (cf. Parker, 2007; Parker, Wall, & Jackson, 1997). According to Carsten et al. (2010), individuals at all levels of the hierarchy hold follower role orientations, and these orientations are important because they can help explain both their own behavior in a follower role, as well as their expectations of how others should act as followers. Therefore, a better understanding of follower role orientations that managers and subordinates hold, and in particular how these orientations relate to one another, could be important relative to leader-member interactions and their outcomes.

To address this, we explore leader-follower congruence in role orientations and examine the impact of congruence, or lack thereof, on leader-member exchange (LMX) and individual stress outcomes. According to theory on the similarity-attraction paradigm (Byrne, 1971; Byrne, Griffitt, & Stefaniak, 1967), individuals make assessments regarding whether they are similar in terms of attitudes, values, and beliefs, and the resulting level of similarity influences affective responses, evaluations of the other, as well as physiological (e.g., stress) and relational outcomes (Byrne, 1997). When values and beliefs are perceived as similar, there will be greater attraction within the dyad, higher trust, and greater willingness to support each other (Turban & Jones, 1988). The affective reaction is thus very positive (Berscheid, Walster, & Barclay, 1969), and the physiological effects are likely to be as well. On the other hand, when a manager and subordinate differ in their values, beliefs, and views about the work at hand, they may experience more negative affect (Schwartz & Davis, 1981), resulting in more negative relational and physiological outcomes.

Similarity, or congruence between leader-follower beliefs is also important in light of LMX research suggesting that similarity influences the quality of relationship formed between leaders and followers (Schaubroeck & Lam, 2002). According to LMX theory, managers and subordinates form relationships over time through a series of interactions and exchanges (Graen & Scandura, 1987). When these interactions and exchanges produce perceptions of similarity in work values, beliefs, and effort, it results in a higher quality relationship (Allinson, Armstrong, & Hayes, 2001). These higher quality relationships have positive benefits for both dyad partners. For example, research suggests that subordinates benefit from high-quality relationships through greater support from their manager, more interesting and challenging work assignments, and increased communication (Dienesch & Liden, 1986; Gerstner & Day, 1997). Managers benefit from increased confidence and trust in their subordinate, as well as being able to count on the subordinate to fulfill challenging job assignments (Liden & Graen, 1980).

Research has also evaluated the effect that high- and low-quality relationships have on stress levels. Yet, most of this research focuses on subordinate stress as an outcome (Harris & Kacmar, 2006), with fewer researchers examining stress effects on the manager (McDonald & Korabik, 1991). In addition, there is relatively little literature on positive forms of stress (i.e., eustress) resulting from a high-quality relationship between a manager and a subordinate. Stress research suggests that individuals can experience stress in different ways, depending on their appraisal of the stressor and their perceived ability to cope with the stressor (Nelson & Simmons, 2003; O'Sullivan, 2010). Eustress, sometimes called positive stress, is a stress reaction that occurs when stressors are perceived to be within our control or within our ability to cope. Distress, referred to as negative stress or strain, occurs when stressors are perceived to exceed our threshold for control or coping resources, or to endanger our well-being (Lazarus & Folkman, 1984). While both reactions are associated with the same initial physiological response, the arousal associated with eustress is typically motivating, and thus leads to improved engagement and performance. The arousal associated with distress is stronger, more prolonged, and leads to more negative outcomes, including psychological and physiological strain, anxiety, exhaustion, and burnout.

The purpose of this review is to present a theoretical model outlining the effects of congruence in manager-subordinate follower role orientation on relational outcomes of managers and subordinates (i.e., LMX) as well as individual stress outcomes for both dyad members (i.e., eustress and distress; see Fig. 1). With so much attention placed on leaders and leadership (Shamir, 2007; Uhl-Bien & Pillai, 2007), our theory begins to explore the other side of the leadership relationship: the important beliefs that managers and subordinates have about *followership*. Our model extends literature on stress by proposing how followers and their behaviors can be a potential source of stress for the leader. Moreover, our relational approach focuses on how beliefs about followership influence outcomes for the relationship as well as individual well-being.

## CONGRUENCE IN FOLLOWER ROLE ORIENTATIONS AND RELATIONAL OUTCOMES

The literature on leader-follower congruence is robust, and suggests that the more similarity there is between a leader's and follower's characteristics, the greater the attraction between the two parties (Allinson et al., 2001), and

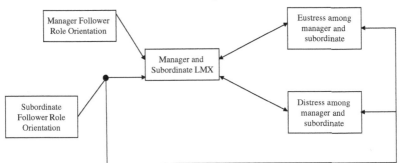

*Fig. 1.* Theoretical Model of Role Orientation Congruence and Outcomes.

the greater potential for positive attitudinal and work outcomes (Hahn & Hwang, 1999; Miller, 1972). Research shows that leader-follower congruence on personality (Deluga, 1998; Zhang, Wang, & Shi, 2012), goals, and attitudes (Byrne, 1997) improves relations between leaders and followers with regard to cooperation and conflict resolution (Deutsch, 1973), integration of opinions and perspectives (Tjosvold, 1998), greater confidence and trust in their dyad partner, and greater levels of mutual influence (Turban & Jones, 1988). According to Berscheid et al. (1969), high levels of congruence between dyad partners increases the amount of reward they experience in their interactions with one another. Although these positive effects have been noted with respect to congruence in attitudes and personality, we seek to extend this work to consider beliefs about follower role orientation.

## Follower Role Orientation

Role orientations constitute belief systems regarding the type of behavior that is appropriate for a specific organizational role, as well as the behaviors that lead to role effectiveness (Parker et al., 1997). Role orientations are derived from cognitive belief structures and schema about particular roles, relationships between roles, and how roles should be enacted (Parker, 2000, 2007). Research by Carsten et al. (2010) identified three predominant types of follower role orientation: passive, coproduction, and active role orientation.

A passive follower role orientation is rooted in traditional hierarchical and position-based thinking about leaders and followers (Baker, 2007; Bligh, 2011; Chaleff, 2003; Heckscher & Donnellon, 1994; Kelley, 1992). Individuals holding this role orientation believe that managers are in the best position to lead because they have more knowledge, expertise, and responsibility than subordinates. They believe that the follower cannot add anything to leadership and, therefore, their role is to "follow-through, and carry out orders" (Carsten et al., 2010, p. 550). Individuals with a passive role orientation would likely remain silent and deferent in their interactions with leaders, wait for direction before making decisions, and exhibit dependence on their leaders for work priorities and goals. According to Kelley (1992), these individuals fail to think critically about organizational processes and outcomes, and as a result, fail to make independent decisions, or take action, without the directive of a leader.

Individuals with a coproduction orientation believe that the follower role is best enacted by proactively engaging with the leader, thinking critically and independently about organizational mission and goals, and taking action to capitalize on opportunities or solve problems (Carsten et al., 2010). These individuals see followers as an important component of effective leadership, and believe that organizational outcomes are enhanced when followers contribute to the leadership process (Chaleff, 2003; Kelley, 1992). These beliefs are posited to drive highly proactive and engaged behavior with leaders (Carsten et al., 2013). For example, individuals with a coproduction orientation have been shown to engage in more voice and constructive resistance with their leaders and to challenge their leader's ideas or assumptions when they believe they are headed in the wrong direction (Carsten & Uhl-Bien, 2012). Kelley (1992) suggests that these individuals think independently and critically about problems, and do not show the deference or dependence on their leaders that is exhibited by individuals with more passive beliefs about the follower role.

Finally, an active follower role orientation denotes the belief that followers should defer to the leader and only offer ideas, suggestions, or opinions when asked (Carsten et al., 2010). Unlike individuals with a coproduction orientation who go out of their way to proactively identify opportunities or threats to the work unit, individuals with an active role orientation engage with the leader only when invited to do so. These individuals see the value in follower contribution to leadership, but believe that contributing without being asked crosses a hierarchical line and threatens to disrupt the relationship with the leader. When asked to offer opinions, information, or engage in some other manner, these individuals will devote their full energy and attention to the leadership process, and can be extremely helpful in solving problems or making decisions.

These follower role orientations are held by both managers and subordinates (Carsten et al., 2010). For example a middle manager's follower role orientation should influence how they interact with "higher-ups" in the organization, as well as how they expect their subordinates to engage with them. In cases where the manager's and subordinate's follower role orientations are congruent, we would expect positive outcomes in terms of their relationship quality (i.e., LMX) and individual-level outcomes. In cases where manager-subordinate follower role orientations are incongruent, however, we would expect the LMX relationship and well-being of both managers and subordinates to be less positive.

## Role Orientation Congruence and LMX

Our theoretical propositions are presented in Table 1. In this section, we describe how we expect congruence/incongruence to influence relational outcomes, that is, LMX, as perceived by each member of the dyad. Consistent with leader-member congruence research (Sin, Nahrgang, & Morgeson, 2009), we propose that when leaders and followers experience congruence in follower role orientation they will experience more positive LMX relationship quality. When there is incongruence, however, each (or both) of the dyad members will perceive lower quality relationships, depending on the nature of the mismatch (cf. Coglister, Schriesheim, Scandura, & Gardner, 2009).

As shown in the shaded diagonal row in Table 1, when managers and subordinates share similar beliefs regarding how individuals should behave in the follower role, we expect them to have the highest quality LMX as perceived by both dyad members. For example, both managers and subordinates who maintain a passive follower role orientation should experience similarity in how they believe subordinates should enact a follower role. Most likely this relationship will take the form of top-down leadership as opposed to interactive discussion or participative decision making (Carsten et al., 2010). In this relationship subordinates are likely to remain silent and deferent in their interactions with the manager, and this will meet the manager's expectations for how the subordinate should behave (i.e., follow without question). Because both the manager and subordinate agree in their assessments of what followers should do, they should experience greater affect, trust, support, perceived similarity and value congruence, and thus, higher relationship quality as reported by both dyad members (Liden & Maslyn, 1998; Liden, Wayne, & Stilwell, 1993).

Similarly, both managers and subordinates who maintain a coproduction role orientation would agree that leadership is best enabled when it involves collaborative interaction between leaders and followers in an effort to advance the mission of the organization (Carsten et al., 2010). Managers and subordinates who have similar beliefs in coproduction role orientation would likely partner in an effective way, share pertinent information, and constructively challenge each other's ideas and assumptions, consistent with Graen and Uhl-Bien's (1995) definition of high-quality LMX.

Alternatively, managers and subordinates who share an active role orientation would perceive that subordinates should assist in leadership decision making and problem solving, but only under conditions where such involvement is solicited by the leader. In this case, each dyad partner

*Table 1.* Outcomes of Congruence in Follower Role Orientations.

|  |  | Manager Follower Role Orientation | | |
|  |  | Passive | Active | Proactive/coproductive |
|---|---|---|---|---|
| Subordinate follower role orientation | Passive | Manager: high-quality LMX and no stress<br>Subordinate: high-quality LMX and no stress | Manager: low-quality LMX and distress<br>Subordinate: low-quality LMX and distress | Manager: low-quality LMX and distress<br>Subordinate: low-quality LMX and distress |
|  | Active | Manager: high-quality LMX and no stress<br>Subordinate: low-quality LMX and distress | Manager: high-quality LMX and eustress<br>Subordinate: high-quality LMX and eustress | Manager: low-quality LMX and distress<br>Subordinate: high-quality LMX and eustress |
|  | Proactive/ coproductive | Manager: low-quality LMX and distress<br>Subordinate: low-quality LMX and distress | Manager: low-quality LMX and distress<br>Subordinate: low-quality LMX and distress | Manager: high-quality LMX and eustress<br>Subordinate: high-quality LMX and eustress |

would be pleased with the more "reasonable" expectations of the other, and as long as they agree on timing of follower contributions, should experience the relationship as a strong and supportive partnership. Managers will be confident to call on the subordinate for help when needed and will not have to worry about subordinates becoming overinvolved or voicing too much (Grant, Parker, & Collins, 2009). The subordinate will feel engaged and empowered but not overly so, as there will be boundaries placed around their participation so that expectations will not be too high. Thus, each partner should agree on the level of interaction necessary to accomplish goals and how best to work together to achieve success, leading to a higher quality relationship as perceived by both members.

**Proposition 1a.** Higher levels of congruence in follower role orientation will be associated with higher levels of LMX among managers and subordinates.

## Role Orientation Incongruence and LMX

As shown in the nonshaded boxes in Table 1, incongruence in follower role orientations would occur when managers and subordinates hold different role expectations regarding the nature of follower role enactments. We expect this incongruence to be experienced as a perceived lack of similarity by at least one of the dyad members (Schwartz & Davis, 1981; Turban & Jones, 1988), and depending on the nature of the incongruence, to have varying effects on perceived relationship quality.

### Passive and Coproduction Orientations

The lowest quality LMX as perceived by both members is most likely to occur when one dyad partner has a passive follower role orientation and the other has a coproduction orientation. Given the strong differences in these belief systems (Carsten et al., 2010), we expect that this combination will likely produce the strongest perceptions of dissimilarity between managers and subordinates (regardless of which dyad partner holds the role orientation). For example, managers with a passive role orientation would believe that followers should remain obedient and deferent to a leader's directives, and refrain from voicing ideas for change or improvement. In this situation, a subordinate with a coproduction orientation who believes in partnering with their leader is likely to become disillusioned by their manager's attempts to keep subordinates silent. Because subordinates with

a coproduction orientation may find it difficult to hold back ideas or suggestions, they are likely to overstep their bounds as perceived by the manager, comprising a relational and/or perceived role violation from the
manager's viewpoint (Morrison & Milliken, 2000). In this situation managers are highly likely to find it challenging to work with these types of
followers because they do not welcome the subordinate constructively challenging their assumptions (Grant et al., 2009).

On the other hand, a follower with a passive role orientation may be
equally disillusioned working with a manager who holds a coproduction
orientation. In this situation, a subordinate would believe that followers
should be passive, deferent, and silent, however a manager would believe
that subordinates should proactively engage in the coproduction of leadership. Managers would likely work to involve the subordinate in decision
making, problem solving, idea generation, or ways to engage in continuous
improvement. The subordinate's preference and desire will be to reject the
manager's invitation to engage, given their belief that followers should not
engage in this way. Moreover, their preference might be aligned with their
ability such that even if they wanted to, they might not be able to meet
the manager's demands. Because of the power structure associated with the
hierarchical relationship (Hollander, 1993; Kotter, 1977), the subordinate
will likely feel pressure from the manager to engage in this way, and
thus experience dissonance in the relationship that causes them to perceive
lower LMX.

In each of these cases, neither the manager nor the subordinate would
be able to act in ways that fit their expectations about the follower role.
Therefore, they will likely have to modify their behavior or their expectations to maintain working relationships with their partner. Because the
contrast between these perspectives is so extreme, however, we are doubtful
they will be able to adequately do so. Therefore, we expect these situations
to be related to the lowest quality LMX as perceived by both dyad
members.

**Proposition 1b.** Incongruence between passive and coproduction role
orientations will be associated with the lowest quality LMX for both
managers and subordinates.

*Active Manager with Passive and Coproduction Subordinates*
An alternative situation of incongruence occurs when a manager holds an
active follower role orientation and a subordinate holds a passive or coproduction orientation. Managers holding an active follower role orientation

expect the subordinate to engage in the leadership process when asked and provide valuable input when solicited.

A subordinate with a passive follower role orientation, however, would not do this, even when solicited. These subordinates would not participate, or provide important information/insight even when asked to do so by a leader. As a result, the manager may perceive that the subordinate is not engaging in a helpful way, and the follower may perceive that the leader is asking too much of them. On the other hand, subordinates with a coproduction role orientation would provide input, voice, and challenge their leader even when they have not been invited to do so. In this situation, the manager may perceive that the subordinate is engaging too much, and is too vocal in situations that do not require their input. Followers may perceive that they are not meeting their manager's expectations and become frustrated with the situation. In both situations outlined above, the lack of congruence, and perceptions regarding unmet expectations, are likely to lead to lower quality LMX for both managers and subordinates.

**Proposition 1c.** Incongruence that occurs when a manager has an active role orientation and the subordinate has a coproduction or passive role orientation will be associated with lower quality LMX for both managers and subordinates.

*Active Subordinate with Passive and Coproduction Manager*
When the subordinate holds an active follower role orientation and the manager holds a passive or coproduction orientation, we expect differing levels of LMX. Given power dynamics in organizations (Kotter, 1977), subordinates are more likely to assimilate to their leader's style and manage their behavior in a way that meets manager expectations (de Vries & van Gelder, 2005; Hollander, 1993; Rahim, 1989).

Thus, a manager holding a coproduction orientation would expect followers to proactively engage, and work in partnership with the leader. When the manager makes these expectations known to the subordinate, and involves the subordinate in decision making and problem solving, an active follower would join in willingly, providing valuable contributions to the leadership relationship. The follower in this situation may be highly satisfied with the relationship (perceive higher quality LMX), because they have opportunity to voice (Van Dyne & LePine, 1998) and participate in important organizational matters (Murphy & Ensher, 1999). However, the manager in this situation may perceive slightly lower quality LMX than the subordinate because they believe that the follower should be engaging, voicing, and solving problems without being asked to do so. If this occurs, the follower may perceive numerous benefits from the relationship while the manager perceives that his or her needs are not being fully met because the subordinate still requires too much management and is not being proactive enough.

**Proposition 1d.** Incongruence that occurs when a manager has a coproduction orientation and a subordinate has an active role orientation will be associated with higher quality LMX for the subordinate and lower quality LMX for the manager.

A manager holding a passive role orientation would expect followers to simply obey directives and defer to the leader. They believe followers should not get involved and, therefore, would not make an effort to solicit ideas or suggestions from followers. Followers with an active role orientation would likely assimilate to this style of leadership, and refrain from getting too involved in the actions of the leader. While this may produce stronger LMX on the part of the leader, however, the subordinate may perceive lower quality LMX than the manager because they are not able to engage in the leadership process in the way they would like. As a result, they may feel somewhat frustrated in a relationship with a manager who insists on doing things in an autocratic fashion.

**Proposition 1e.** Incongruence that occurs when a manager has a passive role orientation and subordinate has an active role orientation will be associated with higher quality LMX for the manager and lower quality LMX for the subordinate.

## CONGRUENCE IN FOLLOWER ROLE ORIENTATIONS AND STRESS OUTCOMES

As shown in Table 1, we also make theoretical propositions regarding the relationship between follower role orientation congruence and individual well-being outcomes, specifically, distress and eustress.

According to similarity-attraction theory, we experience both relational and physiological outcomes when we have repeated interactions with individuals we perceive as being similar or different (Berscheid et al., 1969; Byrne, 1997; Schwartz & Davis, 1981). Physiological reactions can manifest in increased feelings of challenge, anxiety, stress, and frustration (Byrne,

1997). Stress is generally defined as a process of responding and adapting, both physiologically and psychologically, to any real or imagined stimuli (also called a stressor) perceived as requiring an adaptive response (Eliot, 1988). The stress process is intended to help the individual adapt to the stressor, and to find a new homeostasis following that adaptation. Researchers have dichotomized stress reactions into both positive (i.e., eustress) and negative (i.e., distress) forms. Whereas eustress initiates an increase in adaptive capabilities, distress leads to deterioration of the adaptive capabilities of the individual, making eustress a positive adaptive response and distress a debilitating response. In recent years, the term stress has become synonymous with distress, making the term somewhat value-laden. However, since its origin, stress has traditionally been defined as a protective reaction, which helps an organism to adapt to new environments or stimuli. As such, under the right circumstances, the stress process has the potential for positive and adaptive outcomes.

Eustress is a positive form of stress that typically presents as a challenge, thereby motivating one to achieve a goal (Le Fevre, Kolt, & Matheny, 2006). Eustress results when the stressor is moderate or when the individual believes they have the resources to cope with increased demands. Eustress is indicated and measured by positive affective states, such as hope and optimism, which explains why it is expected to lead to increased levels of motivation, engagement, and commitment (Nelson & Simmons, 2003; O'Sullivan, 2010). To date, however, there is relatively little empirical research on the concept of *eustress*. Although many studies examine variance in stress reactions, most research conceptualizes and measures only stress in its negative form of *"distress."*

Distress is a maladaptive response to a stressor; it occurs when the individual perceives the demands are too great to overcome. It is indicated and measured by negative psychological states (e.g., anxiety, anger, frustration). According to Lazarus and Folkman (1984), psychological stress requires a judgment that demands exceed an individual's resources for managing them. In other words, if an individual appraises a demand as threatening or harmful, it will generate a negative stress response (Kupriyanov & Zhdanov, 2014). Prolonged exposure to negative threats can result in physical and psychological strain, producing pathological symptoms and burnout (Nelson & Cooper, 2005).

When considering the link between follower role orientation congruence and stress, both the strength of the stressor and the appraisal of cognitive mechanisms to deal with it become important. First, in cases of role orientation congruence, managers and subordinates have matching beliefs and expectations, and we would expect the need for adaptation and change to be zero or small. In other words, there is little or no need to change or "adapt" one's beliefs or expectations in order to perform together effectively. Their appraisal of stress will thus be low, and the outcomes of congruence are not likely to result in distress. Conversely, incongruence in role orientation will likely generate greater discomfort and require dyad members to adapt their behavior. The appraisal of the stressor in this situation will be greater and result in more negative outcomes. Thus, as discussed below, the degree to which managers and subordinates experience stress, and the type of stress they experience, will vary depending on the nature of congruence or incongruence in their role orientations.

## Role Orientation Congruence and Eustress

Similar to our propositions regarding the positive effects of congruence on LMX, we also propose that manager-subordinate congruence in follower role orientations will generally lead to eustress in most cases, or a neutral effect on stress in others. Specifically, we expect that the most positive effects of eustress will occur when both managers and subordinates share a coproduction role orientation. In these situations both parties will perceive that high levels of involvement and engagement in the leadership process produce more effective outcomes. Each partner will challenge the other to think critically about problems, issues, or opportunities (Kelley, 1992). They will seek creative and innovate answers and results, and look for ways to challenge the status quo and produce positive change (Carsten et al., 2010). Thus they would support and encourage one another in these endeavors. While we note that there is a risk of eustress leading to distress because of the increased work load (Harris & Kacmar, 2006) and the higher level of engagement, as we describe in our mediating hypothesis below, we also expect the quality of the relationship to buffer these negative pressures and provide greater rewards for working together in a productive way.

Similarly, we expect eustress to result from congruence in manager and subordinate role orientations that are active in nature. When both dyad members believe that followers should engage in the leadership process when asked, it opens the door for opportunities with respect to partnership, joint decision making, and innovative solutions to problems (Carsten et al., 2010). At the same time, the belief that engagement should occur through solicitation of input safeguards both parties from overexerting themselves in the leadership relationship. In this scenario, subordinates would be challenged to think independently and critically about problems, and managers would find the unique perspective of subordinates helpful when they face a difficult problem.

Finally, congruence that occurs when managers and subordinates share a passive follower role orientation is expected to produce neither eustress nor distress. In this relationship, the manager's expectations that subordinates will defer and obey are met by the subordinate, however, little or no engagement or interaction is required to produce the positive forms of challenge and motivation that characterize eustress. Both parties are getting what they want from the relationship, and both are meeting expectations for their respective roles. Hence, the actual relationship and interactions between the manager and subordinate are not likely to produce high levels of either eustress or distress.

**Proposition 2a.** Higher levels of congruence in coproduction and active role orientations will be associated with higher levels of eustress among managers and subordinates.

### Role Orientation Incongruence and Distress

When managers and subordinates hold different role orientations, higher levels of distress should result. Research on the similarity-attraction theory suggests that when dyad partners perceive high levels of dissimilarity in beliefs and values, they experience less candor in the relationship (Lott & Lott, 1965), lower agreement on goals (Schwartz & Davis, 1981), and greater anxiety and frustration with their dyad partner (Byrne, 1997). This presents challenges for working together effectively, and may place increasing demands on both the manager and subordinate. When increasing demands are perceived as threatening, and individuals lack the ability to cope or adapt, we expect greater distress for both managers and subordinates.

*Passive and Coproduction Orientations*
The highest levels of distress are likely to result from a situation where managers and subordinates hold incongruent coproduction and passive role orientations. A manager with a coproduction role orientation would expect the subordinate to engage in proactive behaviors that help advance the leadership process. When paired with a subordinate who holds a passive role orientation, both parties are likely to experience greater anxiety and frustration. Managers would be frustrated by a subordinate who is not engaged, does not work to solve problems on their own, or who fails to

speak up with helpful information. Subordinates would be frustrated by a manager's request for collaboration, when the subordinate would prefer to simply follow directives.

A manager with a passive role orientation would expect subordinates to follow orders and remain silent, whereas a subordinate with a coproduction orientation would prefer to be engaged and involved. The subordinate in this case may feel anxiety because they are not able to act in accordance with their role beliefs (i.e., cognitive dissonance), and may feel as though important opportunities are being overlooked by a leader who discourages collaboration. The manager in this scenario would likely feel as though the proactive subordinate is overstepping bounds (i.e., acting outside of role expectations), and attempting to get involved in matters that should not be their concern. Managers may not only feel increased pressure, but even threatened by an over-zealous follower who believes that leadership should be a joint effort.

**Proposition 2b.** Incongruence between passive and coproduction role orientations will be associated with the highest levels of manager and subordinate distress.

*Active Manager with Passive and Coproduction Subordinates*
Distress may also result when a manager holds an active follower role orientation and the subordinate holds a coproduction or passive role orientation. A manager with an active role orientation would expect followers to simply follow orders, but also engage in voice and collaboration when asked. When paired with a subordinate who holds a coproduction orientation, both partners may experience more distress. The manager in this case may become frustrated by a follower who gets involved without being asked, and the subordinate may have anxiety about not being involved in the leadership process to the extent they feel is necessary. Conversely, when the manager holds an active role orientation and the follower holds a passive role orientation, similar results may occur. The manager would expect the subordinate to engage and interact when needed, but the subordinate may perceive that this behavior is outside of their role obligations. The manager is likely to feel isolated without the assistance of the subordinate; adding to the demands they feel in their role (Menon & Akhilesh, 1994). The subordinate, on the other hand, may feel that undue pressure is being placed on them to make decisions or solve problems that they believe is outside their purview.

**Proposition 2c.** Incongruence that occurs when a manager has an active role orientation and the subordinate has a coproduction or passive role orientation will be associated with higher levels of distress for the manager and subordinate.

*Active Subordinate with a Passive and Coproduction Manager*
Unlike the scenarios outlined above, incongruence that occurs when the manager has a coproduction orientation and the subordinate holds an active role orientation may actually produce differing stress results for the manager and subordinate. Managers with a coproduction orientation expect followers to proactively engage in the leadership process, and would encourage high levels of collaboration and partnership among followers. For a follower with an active role orientation, this translates into higher levels of voice and contribution − behaviors that are likely to present challenging opportunities to drive the efforts of the work unit (Morrison & Phelps, 1999; Van Dyne & LePine, 1998). As a result, the subordinate in this situation may experience eustress because of the increased challenge and motivation that is incited by their manager. The manager, on the other hand, may find that the subordinate is not proactive enough and does not fully meet their coproduction expectations because they are not working independently to identify and solve problems, or make proposals for change outside of the manager's request. Thus, while the subordinate may experience eustress from the leadership relationship, the manager is likely to feel distress over the fact that their expectations for the follower role are not fully materializing.

**Proposition 2d.** Incongruence that occurs when a manager has a coproduction orientation and a subordinate has an active role orientation will be associated with higher levels of eustress for the subordinate, and higher levels of distress for the manager.

Finally, incongruence that results from a manager with a passive role orientation and a subordinate with an active role orientation is expected to only affect the distress of the subordinate. Managers with a passive role orientation expect that subordinates will silently defer and obey directives. A follower with an active role orientation will do just that, however, their belief is that leadership produces better results when there is engagement by both parties (Carsten et al., 2010). The subordinate would thus expect to be involved in some level of decision making or problem solving, and want to help their leader in important ways. However, a manager with a passive role orientation may not solicit such involvement, and would likely leave the subordinate feeling frustrated by their inability to fully enact their role. In these situations, we do not expect the lack of congruence to affect stress levels of the manager, however we do expect that subordinates would experience higher levels of distress from the lack of congruence.

**Proposition 2e.** Incongruence that occurs when a manager has a passive role orientation and a subordinate has an active role orientation will be associated with higher levels of distress for the subordinate.

# LMX AS A MEDIATOR AND OUTCOME OF STRESS: THE RECIPROCAL RELATIONSHIP

The LMX literature suggests that the quality of the relationship between a manager and a subordinate may be considered a source of stress for subordinates (Harris & Kacmar, 2006; Skakon, Nielsen, Borg, & Guzman, 2010). When LMX is low, subordinates experience greater role stressors, lower amounts of communication with their supervisor, and more ambiguity in their role (Snyder & Bruning, 1985). When LMX is high, we could expect higher levels of subordinate eustress resulting from more challenging work assignments and more input in the decision-making process. Thus, we expect LMX to partially mediate the relationship between role orientation congruence and stress outcomes for managers and subordinates. However, we also expect a reciprocal relationship between LMX and stress such that LMX will impact stress, but stress will subsequently impact the quality of relationship experienced by managers and subordinates.

*LMX as a Partial Mediator*

Our theoretical model proposes that congruence will affect stress directly as well as indirectly through LMX. The quality of the LMX relationship that exists as a result of role orientation congruence can serve as a facilitator for either eustress or distress. When managers and subordinates are congruent in their role orientations, they experience positive working relations and greater rewards from the relationship that can heighten motivation and engagement (Gerstner & Day, 1997). The resulting eustress from this relationship is a function of their ability to trust one another and their cooperative abilities to advance organizational outcomes (Byrne, 1997). Regardless of whether this relationship is a result of either active or coproduction role orientations between the manager and subordinate, the higher levels of eustress are likely the result of the positive LMX relationship that is fostered by congruence.

One potential challenge of higher LMX resulting from congruence in coproduction orientations is the likelihood that eustress may lead to distress (i.e., a curvilinear relationship, see Harris & Kacmar, 2006). Research suggests that distress occurs when individuals feel as though they cannot manage the multiple demands in their work environment (Edwards, 1996). When these work demands are seen as potential threats, distress may occur. For a dyad that shares a coproduction orientation, the high levels of LMX may result in the subordinate receiving high-level work assignments, greater frequency of projects and tasks, and more responsibility for quality work output (Harris & Kacmar, 2006). If these demands exceed normal capacity levels, the subordinate may become threatened by the inability to perform at expected levels.

When incongruence occurs between manager and subordinate role orientations, we expect lower quality LMX relationships and more distress. The lower quality LMX relationships are a product of the differences that exist between manager and subordinate beliefs about the best way to enact the follower role. In this situation, managers may experience lower levels of trust and respect for their subordinate because they perceive that the subordinate is not acting as a follower should (Liden et al., 1993). This lack of trust may cause the manager to lose confidence in the ability of the subordinate, thus increasing work demands for the manager. Indeed, research suggests that approximately 15% of the stress that managers experience comes from "managing others," and the greatest levels of this stress are associated with managing subordinates that are not liked or trusted (Menon & Akhilesh, 1994). Thus, the low-quality LMX relationships that result from incongruent role orientations are likely to affect distress in negative ways.

For the subordinate, incongruence in role orientations also translates into lower quality LMX. Research suggests that low-quality LMX relationships increase role stress due to lack of communication and clarity around role expectations and lack of participation in the leadership process (Nelson, Basu, & Purdie, 1998). Subordinates who perceive dissimilarity in their own and their manager's expectations for the follower role may experience heightened feelings of role stress because they do not trust their manager and cannot enact their role the way they see fit. For followers with a coproduction orientation, the low-quality LMX relationship may result in negative backlash from a leader who does not appreciate their contribution and voice (Grant et al., 2009). Indeed, the lower levels of LMX would translate into less support for the subordinate, and more confusion and ambiguity around their role.

**Proposition 3.** LMX will partially mediate the relationship between role orientation congruence and stress among managers and subordinates.

*Reciprocal Relationship between LMX and Stress*

Just as LMX is posited to influence stress, we also propose a reciprocal relationship whereby stress also affects LMX. Manager and subordinate stress is a product of both congruence in role orientations and the quality of their LMX relationship. However, heightened levels of stress may also have an effect on LMX. For individuals who experience more distress from working relationships, prolonged interactions and prolonged stress may lead to a sense of burnout in the relationship (Thomas & Lankau, 2009). As managers and subordinates begin to feel emotional exhaustion from working with their dyad partner, it may in turn have a negative effect on the quality of their LMX relationship.

Research suggests that prolonged exposure to strain and stressors can have an effect on the quality of relationships with others (Fernet, Gagné, & Austin, 2010). Specifically, as burnout begins to set in there is a "dehumanizing" effect where individuals find it difficult to relate to others, empathize with others, and feel emotions in an appropriate way (Maslach, 2003). When the burnout results from prolonged stress with a particular individual, these effects may be more severe and more directly targeted at the perceived source of the stress (Stanley, 2004). As a result, we would expect even more negativity in the LMX relationship between a manager and a subordinate when distress levels are high.

For managers, this means that the distress they experience as a result of incongruent role orientations would translate into lower LMX. The lack of similarity that is perceived between the beliefs of the manager and subordinate would produce more distress, more negative affect, and lower satisfaction with the subordinate (Byrne, 1998; Murphy & Ensher, 1999). As a result, we may expect the increased amount of strain to manifest in lower trust, confidence, and loyalty between the manager and subordinate. When a manager does not trust their subordinate or loses confidence in the subordinate's ability to support the efforts of the work unit in a productive way, the overall quality of relationship perceived by the manager is likely to diminish.

For subordinates, the stress they experience from incongruent role orientations may similarly diminish their perception that the manager would support them or stand up for them when necessary. The subordinate may also experience negative affect associated with stress that can translate into distrust for their manager. Overall, the lack of similarity, and the stress it produces, would likely affect the relationship in negative ways, and prolonged exposure to stress may produce burnout in the relationship between manager and subordinate.

**Proposition 4.** Stress will have a reciprocal relationship with LMX such that higher levels of distress are associated with lower LMX, and higher levels of eustress are associated with higher LMX for managers and subordinates.

# CONCLUSION

Compared to leadership, research on followership is just beginning. While researchers have intensively studied the nature of the leadership role and its impact on followers and work outcomes, we know much less about the follower role and its impact on leader and organizational outcomes. A caution flag has been raised in followership research, however, that we should not err in our attempts to redress the lack of attention to followership in overly leader-centric research by swaying too far to a follower-centric approach (Shamir, 2007). In this chapter we avoid this problem by adopting a relational view that considers *both* leader and follower perspectives and outcomes. This view brings a new perspective to the importance of the follower role in the leadership process, and describes how beliefs about follower role enactments can influence both relationship (LMX) and individual-level well-being outcomes (eustress and distress).

# REFERENCES

Allinson, C. W., Armstrong, S. J., & Hayes, J. (2001). The effects of cognitive style on leader-member exchange: A study of manager-subordinate dyads. *Journal of Occupational and Organizational Psychology, 74*(2), 201–220.

Baker, S. D. (2007). Followership. *Journal of Leadership and Organizational Studies, 14*(1), 50–60.

Berscheid, E., Walster, E., & Barclay, A. (1969). Effect of time on tendency to compensate a victim. *Psychological Reports, 25*(2), 431–436.

Bligh, M. C. (2011). Followership and follower-centered approaches. In A. Bryman, K. Grint, B. Jackson, M. Uhl-Bien, & D. Collinson (Eds.), *The Sage handbook of leadership* (pp. 1180–1216). London: Sage Publications.

Byrne, D. (1971). *The attraction paradigm.* New York, NY: Academic Press.

Byrne, D. (1997). An overview (and underview) of research and theory within the attraction paradigm. *Journal of Social and Personal Relationships, 14*(3), 417–431.

Byrne, D., Griffitt, W., & Stefaniak, D. (1967). Attraction and similarity of personality characteristics. *Journal of Personality and Social Psychology, 5*(1), 82–90.

Byrne, D. S. (1998). *Complexity theory and the social sciences: An introduction.* London: Psychology Press.

Carsten, M. K., & Uhl-Bien, M. (2012). Follower beliefs in the co-production of leadership: Examining upward communication and the moderating role of context. *Zeitschrift Fur Psychologie [Journal of Psychology]*, *220*(4), 210–220.

Carsten, M. K., Uhl-Bien, M., & Jayawickrema, A. (2013). Reversing the lens in leadership research: Investigating follower role orientations and leader outcomes. Paper presented at the annual conference for the Southern Management Association, New Orleans, LA.

Carsten, M. K., Uhl-Bien, M., West, B. J., Patera, J. L., & McGregor, R. (2010). Exploring social constructions of followership: A qualitative study. *The Leadership Quarterly*, *21*(3), 543–562.

Chaleff, I. (2003). *The courageous follower: Standing up to and for our leaders* (2nd ed.). San Francisco, CA: Berrett-Koehler Publishing.

Coglister, C. C., Schriesheim, C. A., Scandura, T. A., & Gardner, W. L. (2009). Balance in leader and follower perceptions of leader-member exchange relationships with performance and work attitudes. *The Leadership Quarterly*, *20*, 452–465.

Collinson, D. (2006). Rethinking followership: A post-structuralist analysis of follower identities. *The Leadership Quarterly*, *17*(2), 179–189.

Crossman, B., & Crossman, J. (2011). Conceptualising followership: A review of the literature. *Leadership*, *7*(4), 481–497.

de Vries, R. E., & van Gelder, J.-L. (2005). Leadership and the need for leadership: Testing an implicit followership theory. In B. Schyns & J. R. Meindl (Eds.), *Implicit leadership theories: Essays and explorations* (pp. 277–304). Greenwich, CT: JAI Press.

Deluga, R. J. (1998). Leader-member exchange quality and effectiveness ratings the role of subordinate-supervisor conscientiousness similarity. *Group and Organization Management*, *23*(2), 189–216.

Deutsch, M. (1973). *The resolution of conflict*. New Haven, CT: Yale.

Dienesch, R. M., & Liden, R. C. (1986). Leader-member exchange model of leadership: A critique and further development. *Academy of Management Review*, *11*(3), 618–634.

Edwards, J. R. (1996). An examination of competing versions of the person-environment fit approach to stress. *Academy of Management Journal*, *39*(2), 292–339.

Eliot, R. S. (1988). *Stress and the heart. Mechanisms, measurements, and management*. Mount Kisco, NY: Futura.

Fernet, C., Gagné, M., & Austin, S. (2010). When does quality of relationships with coworkers predict burnout over time? The moderating role of work motivation. *Journal of Organizational Behavior*, *31*(8), 1163–1180.

Gerstner, C. R., & Day, D. V. (1997). Meta-analytic review of leader–member exchange theory: Correlates and construct issues. *Journal of Applied Psychology*, *82*(6), 827.

Graen, G. B., & Uhl-Bien, M. (1995). Relationship-based approach to leadership: Development of a leader-member exchange (LMX) theory of leadership over 25 years: Applying a multi-level multi-domain perspective. *Leadership Quarterly*, *6*, 219–247.

Grant, A. M., Parker, S., & Collins, C. (2009). Getting credit for proactive behavior: Supervisor reactions depend on what you value and how you feel. *Personnel Psychology*, *62*(1), 31–55.

Graen, G. B., & Scandura, T. A. (1987). Toward a psychology of dyadic organizing. *Research in Organizational Behavior*, *9*, 175–208.

Hahn, D., & Hwang, S. (1999). Test of similarity-attraction hypothesis in group performance situation. *Korean Journal of Social and Personality Psychology*, *13*(1), 255–275.

Harris, K. J., & Kacmar, K. M. (2006). Too much of a good thing: The curvilinear effect of leader-member exchange on stress. *The Journal of Social Psychology*, *146*(1), 65–84.

Heckscher, C., & Donnellon, A. (Eds.) (1994). *The post-bureaucratic organization: New perspectives on organizational change.* Thousand Oaks, CA: Sage.

Hollander, E. P. (1993). Legitimacy, power, and influence: A perspective on relational features of leadership. In M. M. Chemers & R. Ayman (Eds.), *Leadership theory and practice: Perspectives and directions.* San Diego, CA: Academic Press.

Howell, J., & Mendez, M. (2008). Three perspectives on followership. In R. Riggio, I. Chaleff, & J. Lipman-Blumen (Eds.), *The art of followership: How great followers create great leaders and organizations* (pp. 25−40). San Francisco, CA: Jossey-Bass.

Kelley, R. (1992). *The power of followership: How to create leaders people want to follow, and followers who lead themselves.* New York, NY: Broadway Business.

Kotter, J. (1977). Power, dependence and effective management. *Harvard Business Review, July−August*, 125−136.

Kupriyanov, R., & Zhdanov, R. (2014). The eustress concept: Problems and outlooks. *World Journal of Medical Sciences, 11*, 179–185.

Lapierre, L., & Carsten, M. K. (Eds.). (2014). *Followership: What is it and why do people follow?* Bingley, UK: Emerald.

Lazarus, R. S., & Folkman, S. (1984). *Stress, coping and adaptation.* New York, NY: Springer.

Le Fevre, M. L., Kolt, G. S., & Matheny, J. (2006). Eustress, distress and their interpretation in primary and secondary occupational stress management: Which way first? *Journal of Managerial Psychology, 21*, 547−565.

Liden, R. C., & Graen, G. (1980). Generalizability of the vertical dyad linkage model of leadership. *Academy of Management Journal, 23*(3), 451−465.

Liden, R. C., & Maslyn, J. M. (1998). Multidimensionality of leader−member exchange: An empirical assessment through scale development. *Journal of Management, 24*(1), 43−72.

Liden, R. C., Wayne, S. J., & Stilwell, D. (1993). A longitudinal study on the early development of leader-member exchanges. *Journal of Applied Psychology, 78*(4), 662.

Lott, A. J., & Lott, B. E. (1965). Group cohesiveness as interpersonal attraction: A review of relationships with antecedent and consequent variables. *Psychological Bulletin, 64*(4), 259.

Maslach, C. (2003). *Burnout: The cost of caring.* Englewood Cliffs, NJ: Prentice-Hall.

McDonald, L. M., & Korabik, K. (1991). Sources of stress and ways of coping among male and female managers. *Journal of Social Behavior and Personality, 6*(7), 185.

Menon, N., & Akhilesh, K. B. (1994). Functionally dependent stress among managers: A new perspective. *Journal of Managerial Psychology, 9*(3), 13–22.

Miller, A. G. (1972). Effect of attitude similarity−dissimilarity on the utilization of additional stimulus inputs in judgments of interpersonal attraction. *Psychonomic Science, 26*(4), 199−203.

Morrison, E. W., & Milliken, F. J. (2000). Organizational silence: A barrier to change and development in a pluralistic world. *Academy of Management Review, 25*, 706−725.

Morrison, E. W., & Phelps, C. C. (1999). Taking charge at work: Extra-role efforts to initiate workplace change. *Academy of Management Journal, 42*(4), 403−419.

Murphy, S. E., & Ensher, E. A. (1999). The effects of leader and subordinate characteristics in the development of leader−member exchange quality. *Journal of Applied Social Psychology, 29*(7), 1371−1394.

Nelson, D., Basu, R., & Purdie, R. (1998). An examination of exchange quality and work stressors in leader−follower dyads. *International Journal of Stress Management, 5*(2), 103−112.

Nelson, D., & Cooper, C. (2005). Stress and health: A positive direction. *Stress and Health, 21*(2), 73−75.

Nelson, D. L., & Simmons, B. L. (2003). Health psychology and work stress: A more positive approach. *Handbook of Occupational Health Psychology, 2*, 97–119.

O'Sullivan, G. (2010). The relationship between hope, eustress, self-efficacy, and life satisfaction among undergraduates. *Social Indicators Research, 101*(1), 155–172.

Parker, S. (2000). From passive to proactive motivation: The importance of flexible role orientations and role breadth self-efficacy. *Applied Psychology: An International Review, 49*(3), 447–469.

Parker, S. K. (2007). That is my job: How employees' role orientation affects their job performance. *Human Relations, 60*(3), 403–434.

Parker, S. K., Wall, T. D., & Jackson, P. R. (1997). "That's not my job": Developing flexible employee work orientations. *Academy of Management Journal, 40*(4), 899–929.

Rahim, M. A. (1989). Relationships of leader power to compliance and satisfaction with supervision: Evidence from a national sample of managers. *Journal of Management, 15*(4), 545–556.

Schaubroeck, J., & Lam, S. S. (2002). How similarity to peers and supervisor influences organizational advancement in different cultures. *Academy of Management Journal, 45*(6), 1120–1136.

Schwartz, H., & Davis, S. M. (1981). Matching corporate culture and business strategy. *Organizational Dynamics, 10*(1), 30–48.

Shamir, B. (2007). From passive recipients to active co-producers: Followers' roles in the leadership process. In B. Shamir, R. Pillai, M. C. Bligh, & M. Uhl-Bien (Eds.), *Follower-centered perspectives on leadership. A tribute to the memory of James R. Meindl* (pp. ix–xxxix). Greenwich, CT: Information Age Publishing.

Sin, H. P., Nahrgang, J. D., & Morgeson, F. P. (2009). Understanding why they don't see eye to eye: An examination of leader–member exchange (LMX) agreement. *Journal of Applied Psychology, 94*(4), 1048.

Skakon, J., Nielsen, K., Borg, V., & Guzman, J. (2010). Are leaders' well-being, behaviours and style associated with the affective well-being of their employees? A systematic review of three decades of research. *Work and Stress, 24*(2), 107–139.

Snyder, R. A., & Bruning, N. S. (1985). Quality of vertical dyad linkages: Congruence of supervisor and subordinate competence and role stress as explanatory variables. *Group & Organization Management, 10*(1), 81–94.

Stanley, T. L. (2004). Burnout: A manager's worst nightmare. *Supervision, 65*(5), 11–13.

Thomas, C. H., & Lankau, M. J. (2009). Preventing burnout: The effects of LMX and mentoring on socialization, role stress, and burnout. *Human Resource Management, 48*(3), 417–432.

Tjosvold, D. (1998). Cooperative and competitive goal approach to conflict: Accomplishments and challenges. *Applied Psychology, 47*(3), 285–313.

Turban, D. B., & Jones, A. E. (1988). Supervisor–subordinate similarity: Types, effects, and mechanisms. *Journal of Applied Psychology, 73*(2), 228–234.

Uhl-Bien, M., & Pillai, R. (2007). The romance of leadership and the social construction of followership. In B. Shamir, R. Pillai, M. Bligh, & M. Uhl-Bien (Eds.), *Follower-centered perspectives on leadership: A tribute to the memory of James R. Meindl* (pp. 187–210). Charlotte, NC: Information Age Publishers.

Uhl-Bien, M., Riggio, R. E., Lowe, K. B., & Carsten, M. K. (2014). Followership theory: A review and research agenda. *The Leadership Quarterly, 25*, 83–104.

Van Dyne, L., & LePine, J. A. (1998). Helping and voice extra-role behaviors: Evidence of construct and predictive validity. *Academy of Management Journal, 41*(1), 108–119.

Yukl, G. (2012). *Leadership in organizations* (8th ed.). New York, NY: Prentice Hall.

Zhang, Z., Wang, M. O., & Shi, J. (2012). Leader-follower congruence in proactive personality and work outcomes: The mediating role of leader-member exchange. *Academy of Management Journal, 55*(1), 111–130.

# AN ENRICHMENT/IMPAIRMENT PERSPECTIVE ON LEADING IN MULTIPLE DOMAINS: THE IMPACT ON LEADER/FOLLOWER WELL-BEING AND STRESS

Michael E. Palanski, Gretchen Vogelgesang Lester, Rachel Clapp-Smith and Michelle M. Hammond

## ABSTRACT

*We propose a model of multidomain leadership and explain how it drives leader and follower well-being and stress. Multidomain leadership engagement, or the application of leader knowledge, skills, and abilities across domains, results in either an enriching or impairing experience for the leader. The result is influenced by the leader's self-regulatory strength and self-awareness, as well as the amount of social support and domain similarity. An enriching experience leads to increased self-efficacy, self-regulatory strength, and self-awareness, which in turn leads to increased leader (and subsequently follower) well-being and reduced leader (and subsequently follower) stress. Enriching experiences also tend to drive further engagement and enriching experiences, while*

The Role of Leadership in Occupational Stress
Research in Occupational Stress and Well Being, Volume 14, 115–139
Copyright © 2016 by Emerald Group Publishing Limited
All rights of reproduction in any form reserved
ISSN: 1479-3555/doi:10.1108/S1479-355520160000014005

*impairing experiences do the opposite. Implications and directions for future research are discussed.*

**Keywords:** Well-being; stress; leadership; work-family enrichment; leader effectiveness

# INTRODUCTION

The scientific study of leadership has exploded in the last few decades, as evidenced by a recent meta-analysis of over 1,000 studies just on leader outcomes (Hiller, DeChurch, Murase, & Doty, 2011), but most leadership research continues to be concerned almost exclusively with work-related antecedents, focal constructs, and outcomes versus person-related outcomes such as stress and well-being. The workplace focus is understandable given that most leadership research is based in the management, psychology, education, and healthcare fields, but the understanding of leadership could benefit from a "multidomain" perspective that includes leadership processes across different domains of a leader's life, including work, community, and the personal life of family and friends. As a key social dynamic, leadership is important in all types of human interactions and thus in all domains of life. The myth that nonwork events have no influence on work behaviors (and vice-versa) is soundly disproved (Hammer & Zimmerman, 2011; ten Brummelhuis, Ter Hoeven, De Jong, & Peper, 2013). However, the study of leadership has largely ignored extra-work factors and outcomes. Similarly, the rich body of knowledge about workplace leadership is seldom applied to other domains of life such as community and family/friends involvement — with the exception of leadership research that uses professional sports teams and coaches as a sample (Katz, 2001). Notwithstanding such studies, the leadership literature has largely ignored what we surmise is a relatively common occurrence among leaders: namely, the experience of leading in multiple domains. An exploration of this dynamic could prove to be fruitful in a number of ways, of which obtaining a better understanding of how such a multidomain perspective could lead to better understanding of both a leader's well-being and stress, as well as followers' well-being and stress is not the least (ten Brummelhuis, Haar, & Roche, 2014).

One way to address the current lack of understanding is by drawing upon the burgeoning study of the intersection between work and life, especially work-family enrichment and conflict (cf., Greenhaus & Powell, 2006; Ilies,

Wilson, & Wagner, 2009; Rothbard, 2001). This stream of research has demonstrated that there are robust within-person spillover and between-person crossover effects, both positive and negative, between work and non-work domains and personal outcomes. Similar effects may occur with respect to leadership, but to our knowledge this question has not been studied in any great detail. We use an enrichment/impairment lens to understand the positive and negative spillover and crossover effects on the individual, which can occur as a result of leading in multiple domains, particularly well-being and stress. Central to our theoretical model is the definition of multidomain leadership engagement (*MDL engagement*), which we define as the application of leader-relevant resources such as knowledge, skills, and abilities from one domain to another. Of particular interest are the conditions under which MDL engagement results in positive outcomes that enhance well-being and mitigate stress and the conditions under which such experience results in negative outcomes that inhibit well-being and increase stress. Thus to consider the process by which MDL engagement results in either well-being or stress, we take an enrichment/impairment perspective to understand when multidomain leadership improves the quality of leading *(enrichment)* and when multidomain leadership inhibits the quality of leading (*impairment*). Further, optimal well-being does not occur from a single multidomain leadership experience, but rather from repeated, possibly habitual multidomain experiences. Therefore, we also describe a feedback loop that may enhance long-term well-being and stress reduction via repeated MDL engagement and subsequent enrichment.

This chapter begins by explaining the concept of multidomain leadership in greater detail, with emphasis when engaging in multidomain leadership is likely to result in either enrichment or impairment. We then explain how repeated multidomain experiences can result in desirable outcomes such as increased self-efficacy, self-regulation, and self-awareness. We show that these outcomes can lead to increased well-being and decreased stress for both the leader and his/her followers. We conclude with some thoughts about practical application and directions for future research.

## A MODEL OF MULTIDOMAIN LEADERSHIP

Most research in the area of work/life balance and spillover (including work-family enrichment) typically makes a primary distinction between the domains of "work" and "life" (Hammer & Zimmerman, 2011). The work-life distinction, however important, may be limiting, and we argue for an expanded view of domains. Perhaps the most well-known research is the work of Voydanoff (2007, 2004, 2001); who has proposed three primary domains: work, community, and family/friends. Within the context of multidomain leadership, the work domain focuses on traditional workplace interactions that are the foci of most extant leadership research. The community domain includes interactions revolving around service to nonwork public or private organizations, including religious and leisure-focused organizations (e.g., serving on the board of a not-for-profit organization or coaching a little league team). The family/friends domain pertains to spouse and parenting roles, but also may include more informal roles among extended family or friends (e.g., planning and hosting family reunions or organizing a fantasy football league).

## The Enrichment/Impairment Lens

There is a competing perspective when it comes to understanding whether participating in multiple roles, particularly as a leader, may have an energizing (i.e., enrichment) or a depleting (i.e., impairment) effect. Within the work-family literature, this competing perspective has received significant attention in the last decade with most empirical work suggesting that both processes and effects occur (Rothbard, 2001). It can also give insight into the stress and well-being of the person. Given that the core research question is to understand the dynamic interplay of a leader's whole life, an enrichment/impairment approach provides a useful lens for explaining the complex dynamics of multiple domains. Such an approach allows us to unpack the positive and negative effects of multidomain leadership engagement. Adapting from Greenhaus and Powell's (2006) definition of work-family enrichment, multidomain leadership *enrichment* refers to a perceived improvement in the quality or effectiveness of leadership in another domain and can positively impact well-being. On the other hand, multidomain leadership *impairment* can be a detriment to the quality or effectiveness of leadership and can result in increased stress.

Most research in this area has attempted to identify either antecedents or consequences of conflict and enrichment (Grzywacz & Marks, 2000) or the interaction between the two (Gareis, Barnett, Ertel, & Berkman, 2009). We know that both processes exist and there may be different antecedents and consequences to both; however, very little attention has been paid to the conditions under which participation in multiple leadership roles leads to either enrichment or impairment and the downstream effects on well-being and stress. Before we address this gap theoretically, we discuss the interplay between enrichment and impairment experiences that result in either spillover or crossover effects.

## Spillover versus Crossover Effects

Enrichment and impairment operate through two different processes: spillover and crossover. Spillover represents a within-person effect across two or more domains. When we describe spillover, we are speaking of the effects of one domain on others with the *leader* as the referent. Edwards and Rothbard (2000) identified two types of spillover. The first deals with constructs that are distinct in each domain but have similarities. One relevant example includes leader effectiveness, in that leader effectiveness is context specific (i.e., effectiveness may look different at work than at home), yet leader effectiveness at home is related to leader effectiveness at work. The second type of spillover is characterized by the same construct that transfers from one domain to another completely intact. For example, mood experienced at work may be displayed at home (Edwards & Rothbard, 2000).

Whereas the referent for the spillover effects is the leader, crossover captures similar effects, but *domain members* are the referent. "Crossover is an interindividual dyadic transmission process that operates when one person's experience affects the experience of another person in the same social environment" (Carlson, Ferguson, Kacmar, Grzywacz, & Whitten, 2011, p. 771). Within-domain crossover effects are central to understanding leadership in that a leader influences the experience of followers, and thus these effects are reflected in most studies of leadership; however, there are very few multidomain studies of crossover effects. Some exceptions include two studies that found that work-to-family crossover effects are present with regard to work ethical leadership and family satisfaction (Liao, Liu, Kwan, & Li, 2014) and supervisor work-to-family enrichment and subordinate engagement (Carlson et al., 2011). Others found that leader family-to-work enrichment/conflict influenced follower engagement/burnout (ten Brummelhuis et al., 2014) and turnover intentions (O'Neill et al., 2009). While these four studies highlight that multidomain crossover effects are real and present in leadership relationships, they also emphasize that the field is ripe for more leadership research to uncover the more complex relationship of multidomain crossover and all possible domains of a leader's life, not just the work-to-family interface. By integrating both spillover and crossover effects, we take into consideration both the individual and relational aspects of leader and follower well-being and stress (Fig. 1).

### *Shorter-Term/Single Episode of MDL*

As mentioned above, *MDL engagement* is the application of leader-relevant resources such as knowledge, skills, and abilities from one domain to another. In addition to a work domain, leadership can be enacted within families, communities, politics, religious and nonprofit organizations, and among friendship groups, to name a few. Therefore, in defining MDL engagement, we are concerned primarily with the behaviors of the leader that assert claims to leadership in more than one domain, and thus, describe such claims as the application of leader knowledge, skills, and abilities. To illustrate this process, we focus on MDL engagement in the context of a shorter term or single episode of attempting to apply leadership resources across domains (e.g., a successful leader at work attempts to lead in a community organization).

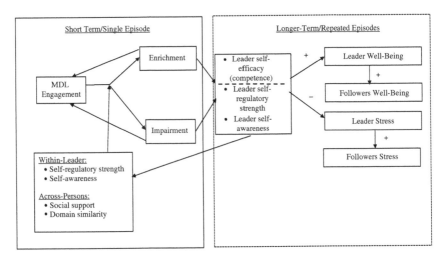

*Fig. 1.* Theoretical Model of Multidomain Leadership and its Effects on Well-Being and Stress.

## *Moderators to the Engagement-Outcomes Relationship*

We have discussed the concept of MDL engagement, and the potential for enriching and impairing experiences to have spillover effects on the leader and crossover effects on the followers. However, there are some potential individual and situational factors that can help to determine whether an experience is enriching or impairing. We now turn toward a discussion of such boundary conditions. We draw from the conservation of resources theory (COR) in our discussion of the boundary conditions of enriching or impairing effects of MDL engagement. COR theory (Hobfoll, 1998, 2002) is a broad theory that informs research on stress, has been applied to numerous contexts, and may be relevant to understanding MDL engagement because of its key feature of understanding resources. The main tenet of COR theory is that "individuals strive to obtain, retain, protect, and foster those things that they value" (Hobfoll, 2001, p. 341). Stress occurs when individuals believe those resources to be threatened, lost, or unstable. When individuals are unable to regain lost resources, they are likely to experience decreased well-being, burnout, and emotional exhaustion (Hobfoll, 2001). Further, COR theory proposes a second general principle that suggests "people invest resources in order to protect against resource loss, recover from losses, and gain resources" (Hobfoll, 2001, p. 349). This second principle is particularly applicable to MDL engagement as it involves such an investment.

As discussed above, engagement in MDL involves the application of leadership resources from one domain to another. Engaging in MDL can be understood as a process that involves the utilization or potential investment of resources. Because of this process, there is a potential for such an investment to be either returned or lost. We suggest a resource investment is returned when engagement in MDL leads to enhanced effectiveness, relationships, and self-perceptions (enrichment) and is lost when it leads to decreased effectiveness, relationships, and/or self-perceptions (impairment). We believe the discussion of a theory of stress (as found in COR) is relevant to understanding MDL as there is a potential for engagement in MDL to lead to stress and potentially burnout under some conditions (i.e., an experience of impairment). It is possible that leaders stretch themselves beyond their limits. Drawing from COR theory (Hobfoll, 2002), we suggest that both individual characteristics (self-awareness and self-regulatory strength) and situational characteristics (social support and domain requirement similarity) moderate the relationship between engagement in MDL with enrichment and impairment. Whereas COR theory directly identifies social support as a moderator, self-awareness and self-regulation are included because they are important variables in capitalizing on the investment of resources for a gain (i.e., to promote effectiveness).

*Self-Regulatory Strength.* Self-regulatory strength refers to an individual's ability to constrain, override, or change responses, whether cognitive, emotional, or behavioral, much like a notion of discipline or self-control (Baumeister, Heatherton, & Tice, 1994). Day, Harrison, and Halpin (2009) argued that self-regulatory strength is relevant for leader development through its role in persistence in challenging developmental experiences. As discussed earlier, engagement in MDL is a process that utilizes resources and can be both challenging and beneficial. Individuals with greater self-regulatory strength may be better able to persist in challenging situations as they have further developed personal resources from which to draw, or may have the ability to avoid situations that they see as particularly depleting. Furthermore, failure of leader effectiveness due to failure in self-regulation is less likely for leaders with stronger self-regulatory strength. Self-regulatory strength can be likened to a muscle that tires after being exercised but can be built and strengthened with practice and with proper rest. Research suggests that self-regulatory strength predicts numerous outcomes such as persistence on difficult tasks, proper diet, physical strength, emotional regulation, delayed gratification, sustained attention, and decision-making (Schmeichel & Baumeister, 2004).

**Proposition 1.** When leader self-regulatory strength is high, the relationships between engagement in MDL and enrichment will be positive, whereas the relationships between engagement in MDL and impairment will be negative.

*Self-Awareness.* Definitions of self-awareness vary, but generally include an accurate awareness of one's strengths and limitations, ability to reflect on skills and behaviors, and an ability to incorporate other assessments into one's self-evaluation (Atwater & Yammarino, 1992; Church, 1997). Self-awareness is a component of authentic leadership (Avolio & Gardner, 2005) and a first step in self-leadership (Neck & Houghton, 2006). It is also positively associated with leader and organizational effectiveness (Church, 1997; Moshavi, Brown, & Dodd, 2003) and is cited as a crucial component of leader development (London, 2002). We propose that individuals who are more self-aware are more likely to benefit from the application of leadership resources from one domain to another. These leaders may be better equipped to apply more appropriate skills and behaviors, as well as better predict how other actors across various domains may react or interpret such behaviors. Further, as self-awareness involves an accurate understanding of one's limitations, leaders with more self-awareness may use more discretion in choosing when to exhibit MDL and may be less likely to over-extend themselves, leading to decreased effectiveness.

**Proposition 2.** When leader self-awareness is high, the relationships between engagement in MDL and enrichment will be positive, whereas the relationships between engagement in MDL and impairment will be negative.

*Domain Requirement Similarity.* The extensive literature around transfer of training suggests a number of factors that inhibit the utilization of training on the job, which primarily revolve around perceptions of opportunities to use newly acquired knowledge and skills (Ford, Quiñones, Sego, & Sorra, 1992). When requirements of two domains are not compatible, behaviors from one domain may lead to conflict and poorer effectiveness. O'Driscoll, Brough, and Kalliath (2006) suggested that a core feature of work-family enrichment was the extent to which work-related resources were transfer-able or exploitable across domains. Furthermore, Greenhaus and Powell (2006) suggested that resources acquired in one domain are likely to benefit performance in another when they are perceived to be relevant and when requirements are consistent across domains. Likewise, we suggest that when the domain requirements are similar across domains, leadership resources are more likely to be beneficial in another domain both in terms of spillover and crossover.

**Proposition 3.** The relationships between engagement in MDL and enrichment will be positive when domain similarity is high, whereas the relationships between engagement in MDL and impairment will be negative.

*Social Support.* The work-family literature highlights the important role of support in reducing conflict between domains and promoting enrichment. A recent meta-analysis suggested that perceptions of support in several forms such as from the supervisors and organization were related to decreased work-family conflict (Kossek, Pichler, Bodner, & Hammer, 2011). COR theory (Hobfoll, 2002), as well as several models such as the Job Demands-Resources Model (Bakker & Demerouti, 2007), suggest that social support can buffer the negative effects of stress. Specific to MDL, percep-tions of support can buffer the negative effects of potential stress involved in engagement in MDL on effectiveness by preventing burnout. Perceptions of social support impact appraisals of stressful situations. The application of leadership resources acquired in the family/friends domain to a work domain may be perceived as stressful when individuals lack the social support from coworkers or supervisors to try new things, promoting positive crossover effects. Engaging in MDL involves the application of new KSAs to a new role. These new ideas or new behaviors may lead directly to increased conflict with others as sometimes innovative behaviors have unintended negative consequences when not supported (Janssen, 2003). In summary, we predict that social support moderates these relationships. When social support is high, MDL engagement will be more positively related to enrichment and negatively related to impairment.

**Proposition 4.** The relationships between engagement in MDL and enrichment will be positive when social support is high, whereas the relationships between engagement in MDL and impairment will be negative.

### Longer-Term/Repeated Episodes of MDL

#### Feedback Loop

The section above approaches MDL engagement as a snapshot, or one instance of a leader's willingness to engage in one enriching and conflicting experience. However, leadership is an ongoing, recursive process, so we now turn to an examination of this process over time. We address long-term effects of repeated enriching and impairing experiences. Engagement in MDL has opportunities for development that operate in a positive development spiral and opportunities for impairment that operate in a negative decline spiral. One element of COR theory suggests that resources aggregate in resource caravans (Hobfoll, 2001) in that having one resource is usually associated with having additional resources. For example, leaders with strong networks are also likely to have more support and a positive sense of self. Likewise, these resources can build over time. By experiencing enrichment (a return on their resources investment), leaders may be more likely to invest in future MDL engagement and experience the benefit from doing so. Alternatively, if engagement in MDL did not lead to increased leader effectiveness, but rather to a resource loss, leaders may be less likely to engage in future MDL. Over time, this may produce a positive gain spiral or a negative loss spiral. We examine repeated enrichment as a positive gain spiral and repeated impairment as loss spiral. We describe these relationships with developmental processes as cyclical and reciprocal relationships that form positive or negative spirals. In doing so, we do not mean to suggest that the relationships are *always* positive (or negative), but rather describe general trends. It is also not likely that an individual would experience only repeated enrichment or impairment, but rather a mix of both. Repeated MDL enrichment may involve impairments that are successfully dealt with, or failures that can be reframed as learning experiences.

Relatedly, as engagement produces increased self-regulatory strength and self-awareness, the increased levels of these constructs will tend to make future MDL engagement more enriching. Conversely, as impairment produces lower self-regulatory strength and self-awareness, future MDL engagement is likely to be impairing.

**Proposition 5a.** Enrichment leads to increased future MDL engagement, and increases the likelihood that the engagement will result in further enrichment via increased self-regulatory strength and self-awareness.

**Proposition 5b.** Impairment leads to decreased future MDL engagement, and increases the likelihood that the engagement that does take place will result in further impairment via decreased self-regulatory strength and self-awareness.

*MDL Experience and Self-Efficacy*
Engagement in MDL through enriching experiences may bolster a leader's sense of self-efficacy by increasing opportunities for practice. Research shows that skill mastery requires about 10,000 hours of deliberate practice (Day, 2010; Ericsson, Krampe, & Tesch-Römer, 1993). Hence, simply practicing leadership behaviors, roles, and responsibilities across two or more domains contributes to developing expertise in leadership. These opportunities for practice may facilitate faster progress from the controlled and effortful processing required in early skills acquisition to automatic processing that occurs when skills are more fully developed (Kanfer & Ackerman, 1989).

The process of MDL enrichment may reflect learning that accumulates over time. Individuals learn from case-based *knowledge* or a schema abstracted from past experiences. A schema refers to a cognitive structure that retains and organizes an individual's knowledge (Lord & Maher, 1990). Derived from one's experiences, schemas shape a person's perception, memory, interpretations of past and present events, and expectations of the future (Markus & Zajonc, 1985). Leaders rely on schematic knowledge to make sense of social and situational contexts (Harris, 1994; Lord & Emrich, 2000). Mumford, Campion, and Morgeson (2007) described these schematic representations as a library that stores prototypical cases. Leaders apply schematic case-based knowledge to determine their actions when encountering a situation similar to the prior case. Further, when an individual encounters a new problem, he or she also refers back to the internally stored "library" of cases and extracts relevant information that can help the leader adapt to the current situation.

As individuals collect experiences, their "libraries" become more enriched, allowing for greater detail in the cases as well as an understanding of the similarities and differences between them. Enriched case-based knowledge reflects cognitive complexity built through a process of differentiation and integration of cognitive structures stored in memory (Lord, Hannah, & Jennings, 2011). Differentiation refers to the number of unique dimensions underlying perceptions in a domain, and integration refers to the perceived relationships among these dimensions (Streufert & Nogami, 1989). This development enables a leader to move from using a general leadership style to a more complex style that is context-specific. By deliberately placing themselves in different domains (and hence different situations), multi-domain leaders force themselves to develop context-specific leadership skills more quickly. Once these skills are established, the leader can expect to have greater amounts of self-efficacy towards unknown situations.

Extant research has shown that self-efficacy is a strong predictor of well-being in a number of different domains (Chemers, Hu, & Garcia, 2001; Karademas, 2006; Magaletta & Oliver, 1999). Self-efficacy is one's belief about his or her ability to perform effectively in a given situation (Bandura, 1997). When this belief is high, there is a positive impact upon well-being (Bandura, 1997; Karademas, 2006). This positive relationship could exist due to the impact self-efficacy has on cognitive functions and the way leaders experience different events (Bandura, 1997). For instance, a leader high in self-efficacy, with a strong belief that they have the knowledge, skills, and abilities to apply to a specific event, will most likely perceive that event as enriching due to their vast resources to complete the task effectively. Each roadblock that comes up during the event is seen as a challenge, which, when completed, leads to even greater self-efficacy. This positive spiral of events diminishes negative thoughts and the perception of stress, creating a positive relationship with subjective well-being, which has been defined as more, as opposed to less, positive experiences in one's life (Lucas & Diener, 2008). Thus, we expect that leaders who experience MDL enriching experiences will have self-efficacy and experience well-being.

**Proposition 6a:** Repeated MDL enrichment leads to a growing sense of self-efficacy, which in turn leads to leader well-being.

Although we propose the importance of repeated enriching experiences above, we also are realistic in acknowledging that failure occurs with leadership experiences as well. Interestingly, some leadership assignments often purposefully include opportunities to fail, because initially perceived negative experiences can prompt increased learning and self-reflection (Day, 2001). However, it is when these opportunities for learning and self-reflection do not occur that repeated MDL impairment may occur. Because repeated MDL impairment represents a loss spiral, it may also represent a decline in leadership competence, or at the very best, a stability. In general, self-efficacy is determined by: (1) signals from the environment, (2) messages from significant others in one's environment, and (3) feelings derived from direct personal experience (Bandura, 1982). Repeated impairment may lead to an erosion of self-efficacy or self-esteem based on negative experiences in each of the three areas. Impairment may occur through a failure in one's environment, such as a rigid or harsh culture, through negative feedback from an important other such as coworker or partner, or through one's own experiences, such as failing to complete a successful project. Over time, repeated failures, negative messages from others, and harsh environments may take a toll on an individual's sense of self. Based on self-consistency motivation theories (Korman, 1970), individuals with negative self-views are likely to engage in behaviors that are consistent with that negative view, which may include withholding effort, failing to engage in developmental activities and learning, and displaying poor leadership competence. Further, poor leadership-specific self-efficacy may give negative impressions to others and lead to lower ratings of leadership effectiveness (Chemers, Watson, & May, 2000).

Further to these arguments, much research has shown strong relationships between low self-efficacy and stress (Schwarzer & Hallum, 2008). When one begins to call into question his or her abilities to handle leadership challenges, he or she may feel greater levels of pressure to succeed, increasing the amount of stress in one's life. When one is lower in self-efficacy, the ability to adapt as conditions change decreases, which leads to the experience of stress (Solberg & Viliarreal, 1997).

**Proposition 6b.** Repeated MDL impairment leads to a decreasing sense of self-efficacy, which in turn leads to leader stress.

*MDL Experience and Self-Awareness*

Self-awareness, in the short-term model, was discussed as a factor on which individuals may differ at one point in time, with those higher in self-awareness expected to have a higher proclivity for taking advantage of enriching and conflicting experiences. However, we also present self-awareness as an emergent state that is continually developed as one comes to understand his or her values and beliefs, strengths and weaknesses, and desires (Avolio & Gardner, 2005). It is thus a relevant outcome of those same enriching and conflicting experiences.

Repeated enrichment may provide opportunities for gaining feedback from a variety of sources and a variety of experiences, all of which facilitate enhanced self-awareness (Hall, 2004). Different situations may call for different knowledge, skills and abilities, and as leaders negotiate such situations, they will learn more clearly about their boundary conditions. Further, an additional source of information regarding one's abilities may arise from the relationships cultivated throughout these enriching or conflicting experiences, and these relationships often play a central role in building self-awareness (Hall, 2004).

Brown and Ryan (2003) found that self-awareness is a key component of psychological well-being and a major factor in mitigating stress due to one's ability to know one's limits regarding one's abilities. Thus, self-awareness serves as its own boundary condition, where the leader chooses enriching experiences that fit with his or her known knowledge, skills, and abilities, and potentially avoids depleting experiences. This self-awareness is not only focused on one's knowledge, skills and abilities, but also the amount of resources (physical health, time, mental ability, social support, etc.) available that may be required for effective completion of the task (Brown, 1998). This self-awareness gives a leader the ability to put a higher priority on his or her well-being; whereas the lack of self-awareness might result in a leader taking on too many challenges across multiple domains, which may increase stress.

**Proposition 7a.** Repeated MDL enrichment leads to increasing self-awareness, which in turn leads to leader well-being.

**Proposition 7b.** Repeated MDL impairment leads to decreasing self-awareness, which in turn leads to leader stress.

*MDL Experience and Self-Regulatory Strength*

As discussed above, self-regulatory strength is similar to discipline or self-control and like a muscle can be developed with practice and rest

(Baumeister et al., 1994). Whereas in the short-term model one's momentary self-regulatory strength acts as a moderator of the engagement-outcome relationship, in the longer term, repeated enriching or impairing experiences can generate additional self-regulatory strength. Through repeated engagement in MDL, these experiences have the potential to build one's regulatory capacity. Because successful MDL involves balancing time, energy, and resources across multidomains, it can be understood as an exercise in self-regulation.

Further, enriching leadership experiences across multiple domains may reduce some of the barriers to effective self-regulation. For example, London (2002, p. 63) highlights that obstacles to self-regulation (such as lack of time, being inflexible in the face of change, etc.) "can be overcome or avoided when leaders take the initiative to apply their own resources (e.g., knowledge, competence, information, awareness) and the organization's resources to accomplish a particular goal." As MDL engagement involves the application of such resources across domains, it is likely that barriers to self-regulation are minimized through enrichment processes. Meaningful relationships, feedback, and flexibility to change also facilitate the overcoming of barriers to regulation (London, 2002), which are all likely to develop through repeated enrichment.

The relationship between repeated enrichment and self-regulation can be understood in a spiral fashion. As a leader builds regulatory capacity, the next engagement in MDL is likely to be more successful, as described in the short-term model. This, in turn, is likely to build self-regulatory strength, inciting the positive cycle to continue. Further, as self-regulation involves the application of insights gained from enhanced self-awareness (Hall, 2004), as self-awareness is developed through MDL enrichment, self-regulatory capacity might be a likely follow-on.

A positive relationship between self-regulatory strength and well-being has been documented in the literature (Ryan & Deci, 2000). This relationship exists potentially due to the increased feelings of control that arise from self-regulatory strength. One often-examined area of research explores time management as a self-regulatory strength, and this operationalization of the construct has shown positive relationships between time management and well-being (Macan, Shahani, Dipboye, & Phillips, 1990).

Alternatively, in some cases repeated impairment can lead to depletion. Burnout describes a psychological strain that results from chronic stress (Halbesleben, 2006). As understood through COR theory, burnout is a longer-term process that occurs through continued threat of loss of resources (Halbesleben & Buckley, 2004). There is strong evidence to suggest that cross-domain conflict is associated with burnout (Reichl, Leiter, & Spinath,

2014), so it is likely that repeated impairment will also be linked with self-regulatory depletion and burnout. Furthermore, repeated acts of self-regulatory failure, such as losing one's temper, procrastinating given unfavorable feedback, or making impulsive decisions increases the likelihood of leadership failures and impairment.

These same issues of self-regulatory failure can increase the amount of stress in a leader's life. Those who are low in self-regulation might feel they have little control over their roles or the amount of work they must complete within those roles. This feeling of role overload is a well-known antecedent to stress (Schaubroeck, Cotton, & Jennings, 1989). Looking at the operationalization of time management, as above, also gives rise to the proposition that those lower in self-regulatory focus will have higher stress. Contrary to the positive relationships offered above, we generally see negative relationships between time management and stress (Jex & Elacqua, 1999), such that individuals who manage their time poorly report higher levels of stress.

**Proposition 8a.** Repeated enrichment leads to a growing ability to self-regulate, which in turn leads to leader well-being.

**Proposition 8b.** Repeated impairment leads to a decreasing ability to self-regulate, which in turn leads to leader stress.

*Crossover Effects: Leader Well-Being and Stress to Follower Well-Being and Stress*

As discussed earlier, multidomain experiences can create spillover and crossover effects. Spillover effects happen within the individual leader — so an enriching experience of finding a solution to a problem at work can lead to additional enriching experiences like helping your child master a musical instrument at home. Such experiences are invigorating and give the leader greater amounts of energy to continue to approach new experiences (Edwards & Rothbard, 2000). Crossover effects describe the impact that the leader's experiences can have on followers, family members, friends, etc. (Carlson et al., 2011). In the work-life literature, findings suggest that enriching or positive experiences can contribute to another's well-being (Beehr, Johnson, & Nieva, 1995; Carlson et al., 2011; Hammer, Cullen, Neal, Sinclaire, & Shafiro, 2005).

In addition to the strong findings in this existing literature describing crossover effects within individuals in dyads, we also draw upon the leadership literature for additional support for the cascading effects from leader personal outcomes to follower personal outcomes. Some studies have discussed how the leader's actions can impact the followers' self-concept (Lord, Brown, & Freiberg, 1999). Others have explored specific leader behaviors on follower well-being (Liu, Siu, & Shi, 2010). We propose here that in the same manner where patterns of leadership can cascade from one level to another within an organization, so can the individual outcomes of well-being and stress (Bass, Waldman, Avolio, & Bebb, 1987).

**Proposition 9a.** Leader well-being is positively related to follower well-being.

**Proposition 9b.** Leader stress is positively related to follower stress.

# DISCUSSION AND CONCLUSIONS

## *Discussion*

The model presented in this chapter is based on a relatively simple idea: how leading in multiple domains impacts a leader's (and subsequently, a follower's) well-being and stress. We have noted that leading in multiple domains, including work, community, and personal domains such as friends and family, is a fairly common experience for leaders. As such, inherent in this common experience are the circumstances under which such multidomain leadership engagement results in well-being and when it results in stress, for not only the leader, but also the followers. As simple as this idea seems on the surface, our exploration of the research uncovered that leadership research has done little to take a holistic view of leading in contexts outside of the work domain and to consider their effects on leader well-being and stress. We did find some evidence of family domain activities on work domain outcomes for leaders (Liao et al., 2014; ten Brummelhuis et al., 2013), which indicate that the need for understanding the role of nonwork domains is important for leadership, particularly in understanding the outcomes such MDL engagement can have on leaders and followers within each domain. However, we feel that the work-family interface can be extended to leadership more systematically and that including domains beyond work and family provides a much clearer understanding of how domains enrich or impair the process of leading. Therefore, we propose a model of multidomain leadership to understand the influence of leading across domains on the leader's well-being and stress and how such spillover can also crossover to followers in each domain, resulting in well-being and stress for followers, as well.

Central to our theory are the actions and characteristics of the leader as he or she applies leader resources across multiple domains. We argued that certain within-person characteristics create conditions to enhance the enriching effects of MDL engagement. Namely, when the leader is self-aware and has self-regulatory strength, the MDL engagement is more likely to be experienced as enriching and less likely to be experienced as impairing. As these repeated episodes of MDL engagement occur and spiral into enriching experiences over time, the leader will also develop greater self-awareness, self-regulatory strength, and leader self-efficacy. As these evolve in upward spirals, the leader experiences a spillover effect of well-being, which subsequently crosses over to followers. Alternatively, when repeated instances of impairment occur, leaders will feel less self-efficacy, self-regulatory strength, and self-awareness, which will ultimately result in stress for the leader and crossover to create stress for followers in each domain.

We note that leadership itself is a social process and is more complex than leader actions alone (DeRue, 2011). Although the role of context, that is, domains, is inherent in our model, we also consider certain conditions about the context that can impact whether MDL engagement is experienced as enriching or impairing for the leader. Namely, we include domain characteristics of similarity of the domains and amount of social support the leader has across the domains to further contextualize the process by which multidomain leadership is enriching or impairing. Furthermore, and noted above, leadership also involves followers in addition to the actions of the leader, and we capture these crucial elements of the leadership process by also considering the effect of MDL engagement over time on the followers who are embedded in each domain.

Finally, our model considers not only single instances of MDL engagement, but also the effects of repeated instances of engagement. By proposing a model with both shorter-term and longer-term foci, we address differences in both level of change and in time. The short-term part of the model captures single episodes of MDL engagement that result in initial enrichment or impairment, whereas the longer-term part of the model addresses repeated instances of MDL engagement and their deeper-level changes over time. Ultimately, these repeated instances result in well-being and/or stress. In addition, repeated enrichment is likely to result in continued MDL engagement, whereas repeated impairment is likely to reduce future instances of MDL engagement. Based on the model of MDL we have proposed, a very extensive agenda may emerge for future research.

## Directions for Future Research

Future research directions may focus on both a conceptual expansion of the model and multiple methods to test the model. For conceptual future research we identify two potential avenues for additional theorizing. First, we have focused on "leadership" largely in terms of leader actions and their crossover effects on domain members and spillover effects for the leader. Future theorizing may consider complex dynamics such as other relevant follower well-being related outcomes (follower effectiveness, citizenship behaviors, etc.), leader-follower relationships, and macrolevel conditions and outcomes (firm climate, firm effectiveness, family well-being, community organization climate, community organization goal attainment, to name just a few). Theorizing may also consider within and across domain agreement of leadership processes and relationship within groups, dyads, or organizations.

Empirical tests of the model provide a myriad of future research directions. Our theoretical model has been developed deductively and qualitative data may strengthen the theory. From a quantitative approach, there are several possible methods to capture and test various components of the model. To measure MDL engagement, data collection procedures will need to capture the leader knowledge, skills, and abilities as they are applied from one domain to another and result in enrichment/impairment. We believe that the complexity of the multidomain leadership dynamics would be insufficiently tested by self-report data alone. Therefore, data collection should include self and other ratings (360 degree or multirater assessments) of focal leaders with data collected in different domains to compare leaders that engage in MDL to those that do not. Such an approach might build profiles of leaders who most successfully engage in MDL. Moreover, research is needed to better understand the types and manifestations of well-being and stress that might result.

Methodology appropriate to the time-frame of the propositions is also required. Longitudinal data collection will be necessary to accurately measure the repeated episodes of MDL engagement in the long term. For the short-term or single episode of MDL, data collection over a long period of time may not be necessary. However, experience sampling techniques could test both the short-term and longer-term elements of the model. In the short term, the comparison of single episodes and their resulting enrichment/impairment and ultimately momentary sense of stress or well-being between leaders could be interesting, particularly in instances where the leaders share at least one domain, such as work or little league baseball coaching. Experience sampling could also test within leader effects of well-being and stress over a longer time period. This research may benefit from critical incident approaches or daily diaries as the short-term theory occurs at one point in time. It would also be interesting to investigate the role of time by examining MDL across the lifespan and across the career. Certain domains may be more or less important at different life stages, and thus engaging in certain multiple domains may have different effects on well-being and stress at different life stages. Leadership may be more formalized in mid-to-later career as the employee gains leadership positions. Of particular interest is the lag effect; in other words, how many cycles of MDL engagement are needed to see effects on well-being and/or stress?

*Practical Implications*
In addition to its academic merits, our model also has several practical implications. The model is grounded in two substantial bodies of knowledge and begins to address a very practical concern for leaders and organizations. From the perspective of the individual leader, our model provides guidance about the role of engaging in MDL in his or her striving for greater well-being. We give guidance about the conditions that bring about enrichment as well as the instances when impairment is possible. From an enrichment perspective, leaders who seek more opportunities to deliberately practice leadership in two or more domains creates an iterative process (Day et al., 2009) in which leader capacity expands, that is, enhancing their leader self-efficacy, self-awareness, and self-regulatory strength. It also provides leaders with an opportunity to reframe their activities in nonwork domains, such as with family and friends, to consider these activities not as depleting but as enhancing their contributions to their organization via their own well-being, which crosses over to followers and mitigating their own stress, thus avoiding its crossover to followers within each domain. Despite this enriching perspective, we also provide insight about when MDL could impair a leader. When certain individual and situational characteristics are not present, leaders may experience impairment, thus resulting in stress and burnout. Thus, creating the conditions by which MDL engagement is more likely to be enriching can serve as a strategy for leaders to manage stress and promote well-being. For instance, building resources such as social support within domains or cognitively framing domains to find their similarity rather than dwelling on their differences, may create the conditions for more enrichment, and thus development of leader resources. By addressing both the enrichment and impairment paradigms, our theory gives leaders a framework for understanding their own capacities for MDL engagement.

At the organizational level, the model provides opportunities to consider how employee well-being and stress evolve beyond organizations' doors, as well as how it carries over to the organization. Organizations may encourage nonwork domain leadership such as creating connections with community partners, encouraging work-family enrichment as part of the organizational culture, or creating time and space for engagement in other domains. Such practices would allow organizations to benefit from employees practicing leadership in more instances than at work and in less threatening contexts for employees to build resources for sustained well-being at early stages in their career.

In conclusion, prior theorizing and research on leadership has neglected to investigate systematically ways in which experiences outside of the workplace contribute to well-being and stress. This chapter proposes a model to meet this need by integrating literatures pertaining to leadership and the work-family interface. Our model considers both a shorter-term, or single episode, as well as a longer-term, or repeated episodes, perspective on leading in multiple domains of a leader's life. In doing so, it offers a set of propositions for future research and practical implications promoting the necessity to consider the very common experience of leading across domains and its potential for increased well-being and decreased stress.

## ACKNOWLEDGMENTS

The authors would like to thank David Day, Shal Khazanchi, and Fran Yammarino for comments on earlier versions of this chapter.

## REFERENCES

Atwater, L. E., & Yammarino, F. J. (1992). Does self-other agreement on leadership perceptions moderate the validity of leadership and performance predictions? *Personnel Psychology, 45*(1), 141–164.

Avolio, B. J., & Gardner, W. L. (2005). Authentic leadership development: Getting to the root of positive forms of leadership. *The Leadership Quarterly, 16*, 315–338.

Bakker, A. B., & Demerouti, E. (2007). The job demands-resources model: State of the art. *Journal of Managerial Psychology, 22*(3), 309–328.

Bandura, A. (1982). Self-efficacy mechanism in human agency. *American Psychologist, 37*(2), 122.

Bandura, A. (1997). *Self-efficacy: The exercise of control.* New York, NY: Freeman & Co.

Bass, B. M., Waldman, D. A., Avolio, B. J., & Bebb, M. (1987). Transformational leadership and the falling dominoes effect. *Group and Organization Management, 12*(1), 73–87.

Baumeister, R. F., Heatherton, T. F., & Tice, D. M. (1994). *Losing control: How and why people fail at self-regulation.* San Diego, CA: Academic Press.

Beehr, T. A., Johnson, L. B., & Nieva, R. (1995). Occupational stress: Coping of police and their spouses. *Journal of Organizational Behavior, 16*, 3–25.

Brown, K. W. (1998). *Emotional body, physical mind: An exploration of the psychosomatic system through the lens of day-to-day experience.* Unpublished doctoral dissertation, McGill University, Montreal, Quebec, Canada.

Brown, K. W., & Ryan, R. M. (2003). The benefits of being present: Mindfulness and its role in psychological well-being. *Journal of Personality and Social Psychology, 84*(4), 822.

Carlson, D. S., Ferguson, M., Kacmar, K. M., Grzywacz, J. G., & Whitten, D. (2011). Pay it forward: The positive crossover effects of supervisor work−family enrichment. *Journal of Management, 37*(3), 770–789.

Chemers, M. M., Hu, L. T., & Garcia, B. F. (2001). Academic self-efficacy and first year college student performance and adjustment. *Journal of Educational Psychology, 93*(1), 55.

Chemers, M. M., Watson, C. B., & May, S. T. (2000). Dispositional affect and leadership effectiveness: A comparison of self-esteem, optimism, and efficacy. *Personality and Social Psychology Bulletin, 26*(3), 267–277.

Church, A. H. (1997). Managerial self-awareness in high-performing individuals in organizations. *Journal of Applied Psychology, 82*(2), 281–292.

Day, D. V. (2001). Leadership development: A review in context. *The Leadership Quarterly, 11*(4), 581–613.

Day, D. V. (2010). The difficulties of learning from experience and the need for deliberate practice. *Industrial and Organizational Psychology, 3*(1), 41–44.

Day, D. V., Harrison, M. M., & Halpin, S. M. (2009). *An integrative approach to leader development: Connecting adult development, identity, and expertise.* New York, NY: Routledge.

DeRue, D. S. (2011). Adaptive leadership theory: Leading and following as a complex adaptive process. *Research in Organizational Behavior, 31*, 125–150.

Edwards, J. R., & Rothbard, N. P. (2000). Mechanisms linking work and family: Clarifying the relationship between work and family constructs. *Academy of Management Review, 25*, 178–199.

Ericsson, K. A., Krampe, R. T., & Tesch-Römer, C. (1993). The role of deliberate practice in the acquisition of expert performance. *Psychological Review, 100*(3), 363–406.

Ford, J. K., Quiñones, M. A., Sego, D. J., & Sorra, J. S. (1992). Factors affecting the opportunity to perform trained tasks on the job. *Personnel Psychology, 45*(3), 511–527.

Gareis, K. C., Barnett, R. C., Ertel, K. A., & Berkman, L. F. (2009). Work−family enrichment and conflict: Additive effects, buffering, or balance? *Journal of Marriage and Family, 71*(3), 696–707.

Greenhaus, J. H., & Powell, G. N. (2006). When work and family are allies: A theory of work-family enrichment. *Academy of Management Review, 31*(1), 72–92.

Grzywacz, J. G., & Marks, N. F. (2000). Reconceptualizing the work−family interface: An ecological perspective on the correlates of positive and negative spillover between work and family. *Journal of Occupational Health Psychology, 5*(1), 111–126.

Halbesleben, J. R. B. (2006). Sources of social support and burnout: A meta-analytic test of the conservation of resources model. *Journal of Applied Psychology, 91*(5), 1134–1145.

Halbesleben, J. R. B., & Buckley, M. R. (2004). Burnout in organizational life. *Journal of Management, 30*(6), 859−879.

Hall, D. T. (2004). Self-awareness, identity, and leader development. In D. V. Day, S. J. Zacarro, & S. M. Halpin (Eds.), *Leader development for transforming organizations: Growing leaders for tomorrow* (pp. 153−176). New York, NY: Lawrence Erlbaum Associates, Inc.

Hammer, L. B., Cullen, J. C., Neal, M. B., Sinclaire, R. R., & Shafiro, M. V. (2005). The longitudinal effects of work−family conflict and positive spillover on depressive symptoms among dual-earner couples. *Journal of Occupational Health Psychology, 10*, 138−154.

Hammer, L. B., & Zimmerman, K. L. (2011). Quality of work life. In S. Zedeck (Ed.), *American psychological association handbook of industrial and organizational psychology* (pp. 399−431). Washington, DC: American Psychological Association.

Harris, S. G. (1994). Organizational culture and individual sensemaking: A schema-based perspective. *Organization Science, 5*(3), 309−321.

Hiller, N. J., DeChurch, L. A., Murase, T., & Doty, D. (2011). Searching for outcomes of leadership: A 25-year review. *Journal of Management, 37*(4), 1137−1177.

Hobfoll, S. E. (1998). *Stress, culture, and community: The psychology and philosophy of stress.* New York, NY: Plenum Press.

Hobfoll, S. E. (2001). The influence of culture, community, and the nested-self in the stress process: Advancing conservation of resources theory. *Applied Psychology, 50*(3), 337−421.

Hobfoll, S. E. (2002). Social and psychological resources and adaptation. *Review of General Psychology, 6*(4), 307−324.

Ilies, R., Wilson, K. S., & Wagner, D. T. (2009). The spillover of daily job satisfaction onto employees' family lives: The facilitating role of work-family integration. *Academy of Management Journal, 52*(1), 87−102.

Janssen, O. (2003). Innovative behavior and job involvement at the price of conflict and less satisfactory relations with co-workers. *Journal of Occupational and Organizational Psychology, 76*, 347−364.

Jex, S. M., & Elacqua, T. C. (1999). Time management as a moderator of relations between stressors and employee strain. *Work and Stress, 13*(2), 182−191.

Kanfer, R., & Ackerman, P. L. (1989). Motivation and cognitive abilities: An integrative/aptitude-treatment interaction approach to skill acquisition. *Journal of Applied Psychology, 74*(4), 657.

Karademas, E. C. (2006). Self-efficacy, social support and well-being: The mediating role of optimism. *Personality and Individual Differences, 40*(6), 1281−1290.

Katz, N. (2001). Sports teams as a model for workplace teams: Lessons and liabilities. *The Academy of Management Executive, 15*(3), 56−67.

Korman, A. K. (1970). Toward an hypothesis of work behavior. *Journal of Applied Psychology, 54*, 31−41.

Kossek, E. E., Pichler, S., Bodner, T., & Hammer, L. B. (2011). Workplace social support and work−family conflict: A meta-analysis clarifying the influence of general and work−family-specific supervisor and organizational support. *Personnel Psychology, 64*(2), 289−313.

Liao, Y., Liu, X. Y., Kwan, H. K., & Li, J. (2014). Work-family effects of ethical leadership. *Journal of Business Ethics, 128*(3), 535−545.

Liu, J., Siu, O. L., & Shi, K. (2010). Transformational leadership and employee well-being: The mediating role of trust in the leader and self-efficacy. *Applied Psychology*, *59*(3), 454–479.

London, M. (2002). *Leadership development: Paths to self-insight and professional growth.* Mahwah, NJ: Lawrence Erlbaum Associates.

Lord, R. G., Brown, D. J., & Freiberg, S. J. (1999). Understanding the dynamics of leadership: The role of follower self-concepts in the leader/follower relationship. *Organizational Behavior and Human Decision Processes*, *78*(3), 167–203.

Lord, R. G., & Emrich, C. G. (2000). Thinking outside the box by looking inside the box: Extending the cognitive revolution in leadership research. *The Leadership Quarterly*, *11*(4), 551–579.

Lord, R. G., Hannah, S. T., & Jennings, P. L. (2011). A framework for understanding leadership and individual requisite complexity. *Organizational Psychology Review*, *1*(2), 104–127.

Lord, R. G., & Maher, K. J. (1990). Alternative information-processing models and their implications for theory, research, and practice. *Academy of Management Review*, *15*(1), 9–28.

Lucas, R. E., & Diener, E. (2008). Subjective well-being. *Handbook of Emotions* (pp. 471–484).

Macan, T. H., Shahani, C., Dipboye, R. L., & Phillips, A. P. (1990). College students' time management: Correlations with academic performance and stress. *Journal of Educational Psychology*, *82*(4), 760.

Magaletta, P. R., & Oliver, J. M. (1999). The hope construct, will, and ways: Their relations with self-efficacy, optimism, and general well-being. *Journal of Clinical Psychology*, *55*(5), 539–551.

Markus, H., & Zajonc, R. B. (1985). The cognitive perspective in social psychology. *Handbook of Social Psychology*, *1*, 137–230.

Moshavi, D., Brown, F. W., & Dodd, N. G. (2003). Leader self-awareness and its relationship to subordinate attitudes and performance. *Leadership and Organization Development Journal*, *24*(7), 407–418.

Mumford, T. V., Campion, M. A., & Morgeson, F. P. (2007). The leadership skills strataplex: Leadership skill requirements across organizational levels. *The Leadership Quarterly*, *18*(2), 154–166.

Neck, C. P., & Houghton, J. D. (2006). Two decades of self-leadership theory and research: Past developments, present trends, and future possibilities. *Journal of Managerial Psychology*, *21*(4), 270–295.

O'Driscoll, M., Brough, P., & Kalliath, T. (2006). Work-family conflict and facilitation. In F. Jones, R. J. Burke, & M. Westman (Eds.), *Work-life balance: A psychological perspective* (pp. 117–142). New York, NY: Psychology Press.

O'Neill, J. W., Harrison, M. M., Cleveland, J. N., Almeida, D., Stawski, R. S., Snead, A. B., & Crouter, A. C. (2009). Work-family climate, organizational commitment, and turnover: The multilevel contagion effect of leaders. *Journal of Vocational Behavior*, *74*(1), 18–29.

Reichl, C., Leiter, M. P., & Spinath, F. M. (2014). Work-nonwork conflict and burnout: A meta-analysis. *Human Relations*, *67*(8), 979–1005.

Rothbard, N. P. (2001). Enriching or depleting? The dynamics of engagement in work and family roles. *Administrative Science Quarterly*, *46*(4), 655–684.

Ryan, R. M., & Deci, E. L. (2000). Self-determination theory and the facilitation of intrinsic motivation, social development, and well-being. *American Psychologist, 55*(1), 68.

Schaubroeck, J., Cotton, J. L., & Jennings, K. R. (1989). Antecedents and consequences of role stress: A covariance structure analysis. *Journal of Organizational Behavior, 10*(1), 35–58.

Schmeichel, B. J., & Baumeister, R. F. (2004). Self-regulatory strength. In K. D. Vohs & R. F. Baumeister (Eds.), *Handbook of self-regulation: Research, theory, and applications* (pp. 84–98). New York, NY: Guilford.

Schwarzer, R., & Hallum, S. (2008). Perceived teacher self-efficacy as a predictor of job stress and burnout: Mediation analyses. *Applied Psychology, 57*(s1), 152–171.

Solberg, V. S., & Viliarreal, P. (1997). Examination of self-efficacy, social support, and stress as predictors of psychological and physical distress among Hispanic college students. *Hispanic Journal of Behavioral Sciences, 19*(2), 182–201.

Streufert, S., & Nogami, G. Y. (1989). Cognitive style and complexity: Implications for I/O psychology. In C. L. Cooper & I. T. Robertson (Eds.), *International review of industrial and organizational psychology* (pp. 93–143). Oxford: Wiley.

ten Brummelhuis, L. L., Haar, J. M., & Roche, M. (2014). Does family life help to be a better leader? A closer look at crossover processes from leaders to followers. *Personnel Psychology, 67*(4), 917–949.

ten Brummelhuis, L. L., Ter Hoeven, C. L., De Jong, M. D. T., & Peper, B. (2013). Exploring the linkage between the home domain and absence from work: Health, motivation, or both? *Journal of Organizational Behavior, 34*, 273–290.

Voydanoff, P. (2001). Conceptualizing community in the context of work and family. *Community, Work and Family, 4*, 133–156.

Voydanoff, P. (2004). The effects of work demands and resources on work-to-family conflict and facilitation. *Journal of Marriage and the Family, 66*, 398–412.

Voydanoff, P. (2007). *Work, family, and community: Exploring interconnections.* Mahwah, NJ: Lawrence Erlbaum Associates Publishers.

# RESOURCE UTILIZATION MODEL: ORGANIZATIONAL LEADERS AS RESOURCE FACILITATORS

Jennifer K. Dimoff and E. Kevin Kelloway

## ABSTRACT

*Employee mental health problems are among the most costly issues facing employers in the developed world. Recognizing this, many employers have introduced resources designed to help employees cope with stressors. Yet, most employees fail-to-use these resources, even when they need them and could benefit from using them. We seek to understand this resource underutilization by (a) drawing on and expanding resource theories to explain why employees do not use existing resources and (b) proposing that leaders, managers, and supervisors can play a key role in facilitating the utilization of available resources. In doing so, we introduce resource utilization theory (RUT) as a complementary perspective to conservation of resources (COR) theory. We propose that RUT may provide the framework to describe patterns of resource utilization among employees, and to explain why employees do not use available resources to deal with existing stressors and demands.*

**Keywords:** Resource utilization; conservation of resources; employee mental health; management; leaders

The Role of Leadership in Occupational Stress
Research in Occupational Stress and Well Being, Volume 14, 141–160
Copyright © 2016 by Emerald Group Publishing Limited
All rights of reproduction in any form reserved
ISSN: 1479-3555/doi:10.1108/S1479-355520160000014006

Employee mental health problems and illnesses are among the most costly issues facing employers in the developed world. In Canada, mental health problems are the leading cause of workplace disability, accounting for 70% of disability costs (Mental Health Commission of Canada [MHCC], 2012), and are estimated to cost the Canadian economy upward of $50 billion annually (MHCC, 2012). In the United States, $150−$300 billion is lost each year due to stress-related illnesses and health and productivity losses (American Institute of Stress, 2005; Sauter, Murphy, & Hurrell, 1990), with much of this attributable to depression and lost work days due to poor mental health (Center for Disease Control, 2014). Similarly, in the European Union, depression is estimated to account for over 135 million Euros each year − just under 5% of the GDP (McDaid, 2011). These significant financial losses are not surprising given that mental health problems and illnesses significantly impair individuals' cognitive, affective, and relational abilities and, if left untreated, can significantly impair individuals' behaviors and performance at work (U.S. Department of Health and Human Services, 1999; World Health Organization, 2004). Moreover, disability claims attributable to psychological conditions, such as depression, are dramatically longer and more expensive than claims due to physical illness (Conti & Burton, 1995).

Recognizing the financial and psychosocial costs associated with poor employee mental health, many employers have introduced services and resources designed to help employees cope with and respond to stressors (Dimoff & Kelloway, 2013; Goetzel, Ozminkowski, Sederer, & Mark, 2002; Irvine, 2011). For instance, many organizations now offer employee benefit plans that are inclusive of services for mental health, such as psychological and counseling services, extended pharmaceutical care, and disability leave (Dimoff & Kelloway, 2013; Goetzel et al., 2002; Merrick, Volpe-Vartanian, Horgan, & McCann, 2007; U.S. Department of Labor, 2005). Employers also provide formal programs designed to bolster employee mental health, such as stress management programs, discounts at health clubs or fitness gyms, flexible work schedules, mental health promotion initiatives, workload management workshops, and Employee Assistance Programs (EAPs). In North America, almost all medium-to-large employers have already introduced EAPs (Merrick et al., 2007; U.S. Department of Labor, 2005) − confidential, voluntary programs where employees can seek referral and/or counseling for various issues, such as stress, work-life imbalance, financial concerns, or child cares issues (Azzone et al., 2009).

Yet, most employees fail-to-use these resources (Linnan et al., 2008; Reynolds & Lehman, 2003). In 2013, the National Behavioral Consortium in the US surveyed 82 EAP providers and found that only 4.5% of employees actually use EAP resources each year. Providers also reported that, on average, they provide fewer than eight counseling sessions for every 100 employees (Attridge, Cahill, Stanford, & Herlihy, 2013). As noted by Linnan et al. (2008), the key challenge for employers is getting employees to use resources when they need them. This is especially true given that the people who could often benefit the most from these resources are also the least likely to use them (Hunt & Eisenberg, 2010; Linnan et al., 2008).

One explanation for low utilization rates is that the service is not needed or necessary. Yet, 1 in 5 North Americans will experience a mental health problem every year (MHCC, 2012) – 1 in 3 full-time employees also report having to deal with extreme stress levels (American Psychological Association [APA], 2007) and even more report experiencing straining challenges, such as difficulties managing work-life balance (Lowe, 2006). Similar statistics apply in Europe (McDaid, 2011; McDaid & Park, 2011). With so many employees experiencing the very problems that EAP programs are designed to help, why is it that only a fraction of these individuals make use of this resource?

In this chapter, we address this question in two ways. First, we draw on, and expand, resource theories to explain why employees do not use existing resources. Second, we propose that organizational leaders (i.e., managers and supervisors) can play a key role in facilitating the utilization of available resources.

# RESOURCE UNDERUTILIZATION

Extant literature suggests that there may be multiple reasons for resource underutilization among employees. First, some employees may fail to seek help simply because they do not recognize that they need it (for review, see Hunt & Eisenberg, 2010). For instance, individuals who are struggling (be it for mental health or other reasons) often have difficulty recognizing that they could benefit from external support or otherwise feel that they are beyond help (Hunt & Eisenberg, 2010). More broadly, responding to any crisis or threat requires, in the first instance, that individuals recognize the need to draw on resources (Dimoff, Collins, & Kelloway, 2015). Second, ignorance or lack of knowledge about available resources and their effectiveness may prevent people from seeking out help (for review, see Hunt & Eisenberg, 2010). Unsurprisingly, if employees do not know about a resource, they cannot and will not use it. Third, mental health stigma, or the negative stereotypes and/or prejudice about mental illness (Corrigan, 2004), can significantly impact whether or not an individual seeks out support and/or treatment (Cooper, Corrigan, & Watson, 2003). In fact, 2 in 3 people with mental health problems report not seeking treatment because of the fear of being stigmatized, discriminated against, or judged by others (Canadian Medical Association, 2013). Similarly, shame or feelings of incompetence (or fear of being perceived as incompetent) may lead employees to try to cope on their own rather than seek help. As a result, they fail to seek-out resources altogether.

Employees who underuse or fail-to-use available resources, especially if they are struggling, risk experiencing loss spirals of decreased health and well-being (Hobfoll, 1989, 2001; Wells, Hobfoll, & Lavin, 1999). These employees may be at a disadvantage in the face of future stressors, and may ultimately be unable to adapt and respond to workplace challenges (Hobfoll, 1989, 2001; Wells et al., 1999). To understand why employees may underuse or fail-to-use resources, we first turn to conservation of resources theory (Hobfoll, 1988, 1989) as a general framework.

### Conservation of Resources (COR) Theory

Conservation of Resources (COR) Theory posits that people strive to retain resources and that anything that threatens existing resources is also a threat to important outcomes, such as one's health (Hobfoll, 1988, 1989, 2001). Resources are described as assets that can help to reduce demands and stimulate growth and development (Demerouti, Bakker, Nachreiner, & Schaufeli, 2001; Hakanen, Schaufeli, & Ahola, 2008), and are integral to maintaining health and well-being (for review, see Schaufeli & Bakker, 2004).

#### Principles of COR Theory
The first principle of COR theory relates to resource-investment − that people must invest resources in order to protect against resource-loss, recover from past losses, and gain future resources (Hobfoll, 1988, 1989). Resources are associated with a cost − an opportunity cost, or the cost of renewing or acquiring that resource (Hobfoll, 2001). Thus, resource-loss is perceived as stress-provoking because it initiates a resource-loss spiral in which employees must invest resources in order to continue to offset past

resource-loss (Hobfoll, 1988, 1989, 2001). For example, an employee may need to invest more time into solving a difficult problem at work so that he/she does not have to ask her supervisor for help until necessary. By taking the time to solve the problem on her own (i.e., resource-investment), the employee is helping to preserve her autonomy (i.e., prevention of resource-loss).

The second principle of COR theory is that resource-loss is disproportionately more salient than resource gain. Although resource gains do not necessarily go unnoticed, their impact is often felt to a lesser degree than resource-loss. In other words, the loss of "Resource A" is likely to be perceived as greater than the gain of "Resource A" – even though the resource itself has not changed. For instance, while an employee who gains autonomy may appreciate the added flexibility, a loss in autonomy is likely to impact the employee more than the gain in autonomy. Given this, it is not surprising that a loss of resources can increase strain and depression appreciably, while gains in resources might not prevent or limit strain or depression at all (Wells et al., 1999).

The third principle of COR theory posits that that the impact of resource availability is even more important when resource-loss has been high or chronic (Hobfoll, 1988, 1989) – as is the case for employees who are struggling. Thus, although resource gain is less salient than resource-loss under normal circumstances, resource gain is markedly more salient during times of struggle. For instance, while an employee may struggle after a loss in autonomy, she will be more likely to appreciate and utilize a new resource (e.g., social support, autonomy in another task, etc.) than if she had not experienced the loss in autonomy in the first place.

These three principles are important to understanding why individuals conserve resources. Yet, they lend little insight into the relationships that they share and the process through which people "conserve resources." Similarly, these principles do not delineate different types of resources or provide much contextual information related to resource conservation. Therefore, it is also important to consider resource-context fit and the role of resource-investment in the resource conservation pattern.

### Resource-Investment and Resource-Context Fit

Hobfoll's (1988, 1989, 2001) proposition that individuals must invest resources to offset resource-loss suggests that individuals must always be gaining resources if they are also using or losing resources. For instance, an employee who has recently experienced a loss in autonomy must try to bolster other resources, such as time or informational support from managers, in order to guard against deteriorations in self-esteem, efficacy, or job performance. Individuals who are using, but not gaining resources, are increasingly vulnerable to ongoing loss. To prevent a resource-loss spiral, some form of intervention or resource-investment is necessary. For resource-investment to take place, employees must first recognize that they are experiencing resource-loss and they must take action to prevent continued loss.

Arguably, employees must engage in proactive coping behaviors to prevent a loss spiral. Defined as the process of anticipating potential stressors and taking preventative action to reduce or eliminate their impact (Aspinwall & Taylor, 1997), proactive coping will help put employees in a position to cultivate resources. In doing so, they will be less vulnerable to resource-loss and will be in a relatively good position to invest in future resources (Aspinwall & Taylor, 1997; Hobfoll, 1989, 2001). Ironically, while employees who are struggling are those who would benefit most from proactive coping, they are the ones least able to engage in those behaviors – subsequently making them less able to recover from the resource losses that they are already experiencing (Hunt & Eisenberg, 2010). We argue that struggling employees will be in a better position to engage in proactive coping if they have access to resources and feel supported enough by their managers to seek-out and use these resources without penalty.

Of course, to be effective, resources and support must fit the context and the problem (Hobfoll, Jackson, Lavin, Britton, & Shepherd, 1994). Applied to employee mental health, resources that will be most effective are those that fit the context of the 21st-century workplace and that help employees cope with the challenges associated with mental health issues. Put more simply, if organizations want employees to use resources, they must first provide them with the "right" resources. Work by Baltes (1997) and Baltes and Baltes (1990) provides an insight into how organizations can begin to invest in the most appropriate resources.

Through their theory on selective optimization and compensation (SOC), Baltes (1997) and Baltes and Baltes (1990) suggest that people try to cope with challenges and stressors by either optimizing existing resources, as they were intended to be used, or by re-investing existing resources to be used in novel ways. Both strategies enable employees to use the resources that are already available to them, such as EAPs, peer or management support, or disability insurance. For example, an employee who is struggling with concentration issues due to high levels of stress may able to engage in "selective optimization" by rearranging her work space so she has fewer distractions from bypassing coworkers or other environmental stimuli. The employee could also temporarily re-set her computer or phone settings so she only receives essential messages and calls, allowing her to concentrate on priority items only. In these scenarios, the employee is using her existing skills and resources to meet demands and make up for her concentration problems.

Alternatively, when an employee's existing resources have become too depleted or do not match the demands of the situation, a second resource strategy (i.e., compensation) is possible (Baltes & Baltes, 1990; Baltes, 1997). To compensate, individuals must seek-out additional resources that make up for losses. For instance, the employee with concentration issues may need to seek-out social support from her supervisor or make a phone call to the EAP if she is unable to rearrange his desk, change her email and phone status, or engage in some other resource-optimizing behavior. Both the EAP and her supervisor may be able to provide her with additional resources that can help her cope with concentration issues, such as a temporarily reduced workload or tips on how to reduce stress and/or improve attentional deficits.

With compensation and optimization, the choice of strategy largely depends on how well one's available resources fit the requirements of the demand or stressor. Given that resource-investment, optimization, and compensation are not cost-free, the inappropriate fit of resources to demands could result in a loss spiral. If efforts do not mitigate resource-loss or contribute to other resource gains, the net effect will still leave the employee in a resource-depleted state. Individuals experiencing mental health problems or other struggles are already in a state of resource depletion (e.g., impaired ability to respond to stressors/demands), and when faced with the possibility of not having any appropriate resources available or accessible, may assume a defensive position, such as withdrawal. Albeit a strategy aimed at conserving resources for later action (Hobfoll, 2001; Tice & Baumeister, 1997), defensive tactics rarely lend themselves well to the workplace − where proactive, problem-focused coping is often required for performance.

Consequently, individuals who fail-to-use available resources, or who do not have access to the appropriate resources, may struggle and reach the "point of no return," where they risk having to leave the workplace (e.g., quit, receive disability leave, or retire) or where they are unnecessarily forced to leave the workplace (e.g., fired or let go). Both scenarios are preventable with appropriate resource-use and social support (Cohen & Wills, 1985). For instance, when individuals appear less than proactive in addressing current or potential stressors, managers, through social support, may be able to help facilitate the resource mobilization and utilization process.

## RESOURCE UTILIZATION THEORY

Drawing on conservation of resources theory, we propose resource utilization theory (RUT) as a complementary perspective intending to explain (a) why employees do not use available resources to deal with existing stressors and demands and (b) patterns of resource utilization. From this basis, we then articulate the role that leaders have to play in facilitating employees' use of resources.

The first proposition of RUT is that individuals must recognize that they are facing a challenge that requires resource deployment. If individuals fail to recognize that they need to invest resources to deal with demands, they may suffer greater losses in the future – hence the resource-loss spiral. Thus, the first key to resource utilization is recognizing the need to access or deploy resources. The trans-theoretic model of change (Prochaska & Di Clemente, 1982), for example, identifies the first step in changing behavior as being "pre-contemplative" – where individuals fail to change their behavior because they are still unaware that a change in behavior is needed.

Employees who are struggling psychologically or personally may fail to draw upon personal and/or organizational resources simply because they do not realize that they need these resources. Individuals may not recognize that they are experiencing crises or engaging in maladaptive coping behaviors. Consequently, they may be unable to access or gain new resources that could help them maintain a state of resource equilibrium – where their resources sufficiently meet their demands. If an employee is unable to recognize that he needs to deploy resources, he will be very unlikely to take action and will resultantly conserve resources inappropriately. This may be especially true for individuals who are struggling with high levels of stress or other mental health issues, where cognitive and emotional processing is impaired.

While individuals may fail to deploy resources because they are simply unaware of their own distress and the need to deploy resources, individuals may also fail to deploy resources because they do not know which ones to deploy or how to deploy them. Thus, the second proposition of RUT posits that struggling individuals may not use resources rationally or adaptively when faced with additional stressors. For instance, individuals may fail to respond to an immediate crisis because they are too focused on conserving their resources to be able to respond to a future, unknown crisis. This behavior is not surprising – individuals are motivated to face challenges in ways that use the least amount of resources (or in ways that seem to conserve their available resources; Hobfoll, 2001). However, resource conservation, while advantageous under normal circumstances, may be maladaptive during times of challenge or struggle.

It follows, then, that individuals may attempt to conserve resources even when they are required to deal with the current situation. The motivation not to use resources may lead to the use of poor coping strategies, such as procrastination and withdrawal, that may have negative consequences in the long term (for review, see Tice & Baumeister, 1997). Procrastination may even be perceived as a cost-free method of conserving resources. While one does not obviously use or draw upon resources when ignoring or putting-off a task, some research suggests that procrastination still exerts a resource cost (Stead, Shanahan, & Neufeld, 2010; Tice & Baumeister, 1997) – a cost associated with allowing a task to "hang on," where short-term benefits do not outweigh long-term costs. By putting-off demands in an attempt to minimize resource-loss, individuals may be inadvertently setting themselves up for more significant resource losses over time.

In addition to inappropriate resource conservation, struggling individuals also run the risk of deploying resources inefficiently – using resources that are already depleted, such as cognitive energy or time, instead of deploying other resources that may be more readily available, less costly, or more easily renewable, such as EAP services or organizational support (e.g., support from leader/manager, counsel from HR).

The third proposition of RUT is based on the presumption that individuals try to exhaust primary resources before deploying secondary resources. Primary resources are typically internal resources (e.g., energy and attention) that are readily available and may be accessed through subconscious processes (e.g., the effect of procrastination). Importantly, for trying to understand resource utilization, primary resource-use leaves no visible "sign" and is not obvious to others – rendering the social-costs of primary resource-use low to non-existent. Primary resources also replenish through the recovery process (Sonnentag, Kuttler, & Fritz, 2010), making them more readily available to individuals. In contrast, secondary resources (e.g., social support, access to tools or information, and monetary compensation/ financial assistance) exist externally to the individual. Secondary resources require explicit external effort to access and deploy, and are therefore part of a visible resource utilization process. Secondary resources may not easily or quickly replenish, and as a result, are subject to depletion and possible social-costs.

Under most circumstances, we propose that individuals are motivated to draw upon primary resources as a first resort and will often resist drawing upon available secondary resources – even when their use may be more adaptive. Thus, individuals often attempt to deploy primary resources before deploying secondary resources because primary resources may be perceived as being more readily available, less costly, and more easily renewable. Using secondary resources to cope with a mental health problem may be perceived as being costly from a social-perspective because of the high levels of stigma surrounding mental illness (MHCC, 2012). For instance, an employee who accesses resources, such as EAP services, or who asks for support from their manager, may feel that they will be perceived as being unsuitable for employment or promotion. Given these perceived costs, individuals are likely to cope with personal or psychological issues by drawing primarily on primary resources (internal resources).

As with any resources, primary resources can become depleted with repeated use in a short period of time. Although this would be a natural point for an employee to turn to external aide (i.e., secondary resources), we suggest that individuals are motivated to rely on primary resources to such an extent that they will persist in this preference past the point of primary resource depletion and may not recognize that this is now a maladaptive course of action. We also expect that this preference is magnified for individuals who are struggling with personal or psychological issues that reduce their abilities to think and act rationally and adaptively.

The fourth proposition of RUT posits that one's health status is dependent on how well one selects available and recoverable resources. If an employee is repeatedly expending time and energy trying to respond to challenges that are largely beyond his control, then he is likely to become fatigued, frustrated, and even burned out. As a consequence, his performance at work and his work-life balance may suffer. While primary resources may typically be renewable through recovery processes, this may not be possible if resources become too depleted. If an employee is repeatedly expending vital resources, such as time and energy, on tasks that he cannot possibly accomplish because of a lack of knowledge, skills, or abilities, then the employee is putting himself in a position for a resource-loss spiral.

In this respect, we echo Hobfoll's (1988, 1989, 2001) sentiments that resource-use is rarely cost-free. To use primary or secondary resources, individuals must engage in resource-investment, optimization, or compensation. The effects of these investments are felt much more significantly when resource deployment has been frequent or extensive. Thus, repeated, rapid, or extensive deployment of resources can lead to resource depletion and exhaustion because resource reserves do not have a chance to recover and replenish. Once at this stage, employees — whether healthy or not — are at a substantial risk for crisis as their resource pool becomes exhausted. As a result, employees who may have been able to rebound from a minor struggle are now experiencing more significant challenges that are difficult and time-consuming to overcome; employees who were already struggling are now experiencing physical or psychological collapse — a point at which they will be unable to recover from without substantial assistance, which they may now have trouble accessing.

To a large extent, this is where early recognition and action are critical. Rather than engage in repeated or excessive resource-use, employees should engage in early and appropriate resource-use. To be successful, early resource-use relies upon employees being able to (a) recognize that they need to deploy resources and (b) select the resources that are best suited to their needs. For struggling employees, this is no easy feat. We posit that managers are not only key gatekeepers to secondary resources, but also that they can help put employees on a path that will enable them to choose effectively. First, managers can help individuals to recognize when they are struggling and might be in need of secondary resources. Second, managers can facilitate resource utilization by providing social support and discussing resource options with employees.

## RESOURCE UTILIZATION THEORY AND THE ROLE OF MANAGERS

In alignment with the propositions set forth by RUT, we argue that managers can play a substantial role in employee resource-use, especially for employees who may be struggling. Not only can managers build awareness of available resources and programs, but they can also serve as a "first line of defense" in recognizing potential problems and/or warning signs of a struggling employee (Fleten & Johnsen, 2006; Nieuwenhuijsen, Verbeek, De Boer, Blonk, & Van Dijk, 2004). In doing so, managers may be able to stop or prevent a loss spiral. The prognosis for mental health problems can be improved through early recognition and intervention (Craig et al., 2004), so if leaders are able to recognize warning signs of deteriorating mental health, they may also be able to help provide referral to resources, such as EAPs.

Under conditions of challenge or high demands, be they work-related or not, employees need to be able to seek-out and receive appropriate resources that will prevent strain, burnout, and/or severe mental illness. Managers can help facilitate this process through their knowledge of the employee and the policies, solutions, and resources at the organization. Managers also hold a hierarchical position of authority, where they are able to discuss issues related to workplace performance and behavior (Ito & Brotheridge, 2003). For instance, if a manager notices an employee is not paying attention in meetings or has been abnormally inattentive to important details, a manager may address these issues professionally and compassionately by bringing these issues to the employee's attention, asking the employee if she/he needs help, and providing accessibility to available resources (e.g., EAP information, workplace redistribution options, accommodation possibilities, etc.), and social support.

Consistent with Hobfoll's (1989) proposition that resources are particularly salient under demanding conditions, struggling employees may be more receptive to resource-related suggestions and support from their managers. Although resource gains may have minimal impact on people who are not experiencing resource losses, gains can become more apparent when significant or sustained resource-loss has been experienced (Hobfoll, 1988, 1989) — as is the case with the development of a mental health problem. Resource utilization, under these circumstances, may have the capacity for broader individual impacts, such as improved health and well-being, as well as organizational-and team-level outcomes, such as improved interpersonal relationships and reduced absenteeism and disability leave. Thus, managers have the potential to improve employee well-being and workplace outcomes by first recognizing signs of struggle or distress, then providing information and access to resources, and finally by normalizing mental health issues by lowering stigma and providing social support.

### Social Support Theory and the Role of Leaders

Defined as "the social resources that persons perceive to be available or that are actually provided to them" (Gottlieb & Bergen, 2010, p. 512), social support can widen an employee's pool of available resources and can replace other resources that have been lacking or even lost. Multiple decades of research findings in the area suggest that social support is one of the most well-known and highly effective situational variables capable of buffering against job strain (Cohen & Wills, 1985; Johnson & Hall, 1988).

Resource theories view social support as a robust resource that can impact the likelihood that someone will experience a resource-loss spiral or a resource gain spiral. The presence of social support can help encourage resiliency, bolster stress resistance, and improve health by serving as a gateway to other resources (Hobfoll, 2001; Schumm, Briggs-Phillips, & Hobfoll, 2006). For instance, individuals with high levels of social support also experience improved health, positive well-being, and increased self-esteem (Cropanzano & Mitchell, 2005). Many researchers contend that social support can lead to positive outcomes by reinforcing positive aspects of the self (Swann & Predmore, 1985), by engaging in perspective-taking that can make the stressful situation seem less threatening (Bakker & Demerouti, 2007), by providing feedback that connotes caring (Heaney, Price, & Rafferty, 1995), and by helping individuals exert control through the provision of instrumental aid or advice (House, 1981; Malecki & Demaray, 2003).

Social support from supervisors has been indirectly and directly linked to employee health and well-being (Ganster, Fusilier, & Mayes, 1986). For instance, social support is thought to indirectly enhance mental health by helping to improve employee coping behavior (Folkman & Lazarus, 1980), and directly enhance well-being by increasing self-esteem, bolstering morale (Heller, Swindle, & Dusenbury, 1986), and providing instrumental tools to help employees perform well (Van der Doef & Maes, 1999). Consequently, social support from leaders can take many forms, best categorized by House (1981) into four primary "social support types": emotional, instrumental, informational, and appraisal support. Emotional support largely involves portrayal of feelings of trust and caring, while instrumental support often involves more tangible resources, such as time, materials, or money (House, 1981). Informational support involves information or advice, and appraisal support is defined as support that involves providing evaluative feedback to others – making it somewhat distinct from informational support (House, 1981).

While social support, as a global construct, has been linked to positive workplace outcomes (Malecki & Demaray, 2003), each support type's ability to function as an appropriate resource is somewhat context-specific (Malecki & Demaray, 2003). For instance, it is plausible that instrumental types of support are especially appropriate in situations that are controllable or that have easily available solutions, whereas emotional support may be more helpful in situations where no solutions are readily available (Cutrona & Russell, 1990; Cutrona & Suhr, 1994; Gottlieb & Bergen, 2010). However, within the context of mental health, it is likely that managers will employ all four types of social support in unison, albeit relying on emotional, instrumental, and informational support more often. For instance, managers must (a) be compassionate (i.e., emotionally supportive) when addressing warning signs, (b) take time out of their day to meet with a struggling employee and possibly make accommodations (i.e., instrumental support), and (c) be ready to provide information surrounding available resources, such as EAP (i.e., informational support).

Yet, according to Barling, MacEwen, and Pratt (1988) and others (Tardy, 1994), people often do not typically distinguish between the different types of support that they receive — they merely perceive someone as being globally supportive. Thus, instrumental acts may be perceived as having emotional implications depending on the situation. For instance, a leader demonstrates instrumental support when he or she works hard to ensure that an accommodation plan is effective for an employee with anxiety. Yet, the leader's effort can also communicate something about his or her relationship with the employee — that the leader cares about the employee and their well-being. Consequently, the emotional meaning of instrumental support can have broader emotional implications.

Still, it may not be so much about the type of support delivered, but rather the way by which it is delivered. For instance, well-intentioned, but unsuitable, clumsy, or overbearing support can be unhelpful and even psychologically damaging (Steinberg & Gottlieb, 1994). This consequence could be especially problematic if experienced by an employee with a mental health problem. Thus, it is important that managers know what to do, but also *how* to do it. Struggling employees who will seek-out resources and benefit most from social support are those who have leaders who are able to match the type of support provided with the characteristics of the situation (Chiu, Hong, Mischel, & Shoda, 1995; Cutrona & Russell, 1990), and who are able to deliver all types of support in an emotionally supportive way (Barling et al., 1988; Chiu et al., 1995; Tardy, 1994).

Leaders who socially support their employees are likely to help facilitate resource-use among employees — especially among those who are struggling. Leaders who are capable of recognizing the warning signs associated with a struggling employee may be able to help initiate contact, provide support, and resultantly direct employees toward additional resources that they can use. Findings from a recent study by Dimoff, Kelloway, and Burnstein (2015) suggest that the initiation of this process may be possible with leader-focused training. Following a three-hour mental health awareness training (MHAT), leaders experienced long-term improvements in knowledge, stigma, confidence, and promotion intentions surrounding employee mental health and employee mental health resources. Moreover, up to nine months post-training, mental health-related disability durations were reduced by approximately 19 days per claim among employee groups whose leaders attended the training. This significant reduction speaks to the importance of training leaders to (a) recognize the warning signs of a struggling employee and (b) direct employees toward potential resources.

The two-module design of the training was reported to have helped achieve these goals. The first module was focused on knowledge-building (Saks, Haccoun, & Belcourt, 2004), with an emphasis on teaching managers when intervention was appropriate. Thus, the training focused on the behavioral signs associated with (a) acute stress and chronic strain, (b) the negative consequences of strain and other mental health problems, and (c) the role of leaders as sources of support for struggling employees. The second lecture-based module was designed to improve leaders' ability to intervene and focused on the resources available to employees and how to access them. Particular attention was focused on the leaders' role as a referral agent — leaders were taught that their role was not to diagnose or to intervene in mental health issues but, rather, to refer employees to the appropriate resources within the organization or community. Thus, leaders were trained in alignment with the four propositions outlined by RUT — to help employees (a) recognize when they are struggling, (b) realize that they can benefit from resource deployment, (c) conserve vital primary resources, and (d) utilize secondary resources that can help prevent a loss spiral.

## CONCLUSIONS

Resource underutilization is one of the biggest challenges facing organizations and human resources departments in the developed world. With 20% of the workforce experiencing mental health problems every year, and with approximately 30% of employees reporting that they have to deal with straining challenges on a regular basis, resources should be used widely and often (APA, 2007; Lowe, 2006; MHCC, 2012). Yet, only 4.5% of employees utilize available resources, such as EAPs that provide myriad of solutions and assistance for mental health problems, personal problems, and even financial and legal problems (Attridge et al., 2013). While much of the mental health literature explains resource underutilization as being a product of high stigma levels and lack of awareness, resource theories suggest that an underlying issue may be more closely related to employees' motivations to conserve resources. In this chapter, we introduce resource utilization theory to help pair these rationales and further explain resource underutilization patterns, in general, and within the context of employee mental health and well-being. We suggest that leaders in organizations have a particularly important role to play in resource facilitation. To further explore this role, we recommend that future research aim to empirically evaluate the propositions introduced in this chapter.

# REFERENCES

American Institute of Stress. (2005). *Workplace stress.* Retrieved from http://www.stress.org/ workplace-stress/. Accessed on August 27, 2015.

American Psychological Association. (2007). *Stress survey: Stress a major health problem in the U.S.* Retrieved from http://www.apahelpcenter.org/articles/article/php?id = 165

Aspinwall, L. G., & Taylor, S. E. (1997). A stitch in time: Self-regulation and pro-active coping. *Psychological Bulletin, 121,* 417–436.

Attridge, M., Cahill, T., Stanford, G., & Herlihy, P. A. (2013). The national behavioral consortium benchmarking study: Industry profile of 82 external EAP providers. *Journal of Workplace Behavioral Health, 28,* 251–324.

Azzone, V., McCann, B., Merrick, E. L., Hiatt, D., Hodgkin, D., & Horgan, C. (2009). Workplace stress, organizational factors and EAP utilization. *Journal of Workplace Behavioral Health, 24,* 344–356.

Bakker, A. B., & Demerouti, E. (2007). The job demands-resources model: State of the art. *Journal of Managerial Psychology, 22,* 309–328.

Baltes, M. M., & Baltes, P. B. (1990). Psychological perspectives on successful aging: The model of selective optimization with compensation. In P. B. Baltes (Eds.), *Successful aging: Perspectives from the behavioral sciences* (pp. 1–34). New York, NY: Cambridge University Press.

Baltes, R. B. (1997). On the incomplete architecture of human ontogeny: Selection, optimization, and compensation as foundation of development theory. *American Psychologist, 52,* 366–380.

Barling, J., MacEwen, K. E., & Pratt, L. (1988). Manipulating the type and source of social support: An experimental investigation. *Canadian Journal of Behavioural Science, 20,* 140–154.

Canadian Medical Association. (2013). *Mental health.* Retrieved from https://www.cma.ca/En/ Pages/mental-health.aspx. Accessed on August 3, 2015.

Center for Disease Control. (2014). *Workplace health promotion: Depression.* Retrieved from http://www.cdc.gov/workplacehealthpromotion/implementation/topics/depression.html. Accessed on August 11, 2015.

Chiu, C. Y., Hong, Y. Y., Mischel, W., & Shoda, Y. (1995). Discriminative facility in social competence: Conditional versus dispositional encoding and monitoring-blunting of information. *Social Cognition, 13,* 49–70.

Cohen, S., & Wills, T. A. (1985). Stress, social support, and the buffering hypothesis. *Psychological Bulletin, 98,* 310–357.

Conti, D. J., & Burton, W. N. (1995). The cost of depression in the workplace. *Behavioral Healthcare* Tomorrow, *4,* 25–27.

Cooper, A. E., Corrigan, P. W., & Watson, A. C. (2003). Mental illness stigma and care seeking. *The Journal of Nervous and Mental Disease, 191*, 339–341.

Corrigan, P. (2004). How stigma interferes with mental health care. *American Psychologist, 59*, 614–625.

Craig, T., Garety, P., Power, P., Rahaman, N., Colbert, S., Fornells-Ambrojo, M., & Dunn, G. (2004). The Lambeth early onset (LEO) team: Randomized controlled trial of the effectiveness of specialized care for early psychosis. *British Medical Journal, 329*, 1–5.

Cropanzano, R., & Mitchell, M. S. (2005). Social exchange theory: An interdisciplinary review. *Journal of Management, 31*, 874–900.

Cutrona, C. E., & Russell, D. W. (1990). Type of social support and specific stress: Toward a theory of optimal matching. In B. R. Sarason, I. G. Sarason, & G. R. Pierce (Eds.), *Social support: An interactional view* (pp. 319–366). Oxford, England: Wiley.

Cutrona, C. E., & Suhr, J. A. (1994). Social support communication in the context of marriage: An analysis of couples' supportive interactions. In B. R. Burleson, T. L. Albrecht, & I. G. Sarason (Eds.), *Communication of social support: Messages, interactions, relationships, and community* (pp. 113–135). Thousand Oaks, CA: Safe.

Demerouti, E., Bakker, A. B., Nachreiner, F., & Schaufeli, W. B. (2001). The job demands – Resources model of burnout. *Journal of Applied Psychology, 86*, 499–512.

Dimoff, J. K., Collins, L., & Kelloway, E. K. (2015). Scrambling: An ability and a process. In C. L. Cooper & A. S. Antoniou (Eds.), *Coping, personality and the workplace: Responding to psychological crisis and critical events*. Farnham: Gower.

Dimoff, J. K., & Kelloway, E. K. (2013). Bridging the gap: Workplace mental health research in Canada. *Psychologie Canadienne. [Canadian Psychology.], 54*, 203–212.

Dimoff, J. K., Kelloway, E. K., & Burnstein, M. D. (2015). Mental Health Awareness Training (MHAT): The development and evaluation of an intervention for workplace leaders. *International Journal of Stress Management, 23*, 167–189.

Eisenberg, D., Downs, M. F., Golberstein, E., & Zivin, K. (2009). Stigma and help seeking for mental health among college students. *Medical Care Research and Review, 66*, 522–541.

Fleten, N., & Johnsen, R. (2006). Reducing sick leave by minimal postal intervention: A randomised, controlled intervention study. *Occupational and Environmental Medicine, 63*, 676–682.

Folkman, S., & Lazarus, R. S. (1980). An analysis of coping in a middle-aged community sample. *Journal of Health and Social Behavior, 21*, 219–239.

Ganster, D. C., Fusilier, M. R., & Mayes, B. T. (1986). Role of social support in the experiences of stress at work. *Journal of Applied Psychology, 71*, 102–110.

Goetzel, R. Z., Ozminkowski, R. J., Sederer, L. I., & Mark, T. L. (2002). The business case for quality mental health services: Why employers should care about the mental health and well-being of their employees. *Journal of Occupational and Environmental Medicine, 44*, 320–330.

Gottlieb, B. H., & Bergen, A. E. (2010). Social support concepts and measures. *Journal of Psychosomatic Research, 69*, 511–520.

Hakanen, J. J., Schaufeli, W. B., & Ahola, K. (2008). The job demands-resources model: A three-year cross-lagged study of burnout, depression, commitment, and work engagement. *Work & Stress, 22*, 224–241.

Heaney, C. A., Price, R. H., & Rafferty, J. (1995). Increasing coping resources at work: A field experiment to increase social support, improve work team functioning, and enhance employee mental health. *Journal of Organizational Behavior, 16*, 335–352.

Heller, K., Swindle, R. W., & Dusenbury, L. (1986). Component social support processes: Comments and integration. *Journal of Consulting and Clinical Psychology, 54*, 466–470.

Hobfoll, S. E. (1988). *The ecology of stress.* New York, NY: Hemisphere Publishing Corporation.

Hobfoll, S. E. (1989). Conservation of resources: A new attempt at conceptualizing stress. *American Psychologist, 44*, 513–524.

Hobfoll, S. E. (1998). *Stress, culture, and community: The psychology and philosophy of stress.* New York, NY: Plenum.

Hobfoll, S. E. (2001). The influence of culture, community, and the nested-self in the stress process: Advancing conservation of resources theory. *Applied Psychology, 50*, 337–421.

Hobfoll, S. E., Jackson, A. P., Lavin, J., Britton, P. J., & Shepherd, J. B. (1994). Reducing inner-city women's AIDS risk activities: A study of single, pregnant women. *Health Psychology, 13*, 397–403.

House, J. S. (1981). *Work stress and social support.* Reading, MA: Addison-Wesley.

Hunt, J., & Eisenberg, D. (2010). Mental health problems and help-seeking behavior among college students. *Journal of Adolescent Health, 46*, 3–10.

Irvine, A. (2011). Something to declare? The disclosure of common mental health problems at work. *Disability & Society, 26*, 179–192.

Ito, J. K., & Brotheridge, C. M. (2003). Resources, coping strategies, and emotional exhaustion: A conservation of resources perspective. *Journal of Vocational Behavior, 63*, 490–509.

Johnson, J. V., & Hall, E. M. (1988). Job strain, work place social support, and cardiovascular disease: A cross-sectional study of a random sample of the Swedish working population. *American Journal of Public Health, 78*, 1336–1342.

Linnan, L., Bowling, M., Childress, J., Lindsay, G., Blakey, C., Pronk, S., & Royall, P. (2008). Results of the 2004 national worksite health promotion survey. *American Journal of Public Health, 98*, 1503–1509.

Lowe, G. (2006). *Under pressure: Implications of work-life balance and job stress.* Vancouver: William Banwell Human Solutions. Retrieved from http://gwlcentreformentalhealth. com/english/pdf/s7_004818.pdf

Malecki, C. K., & Demaray, M. K. (2003). What type of support do they need? Investigating student adjustment as related to emotional, informational, appraisal, and instrumental support. *School Psychology Quarterly, 18*, 231–252.

McDaid, D. (2011). *Making the long-term economic case for investing in mental health to contribute to sustainability.* European Union. Retrieved from http://ec.europa.eu/health/mental_health/docs/long_term_sustainability_en.pdf

McDaid, D., & Park, A. (2011). *Investing in mental health and wellbeing: Findings from the DataPREV project.* London: London School of Economics.

Mental Health Commission of Canada. (2012). *Changing directions, changing lives: The mental health strategy for Canada.* Calgary, AB: Mental Health Commission of Canada.

Merrick, E. S. L., Volpe-Vartanian, J., Horgan, C. M., & McCann, B. (2007). Revisiting employee assistance programs and substance use problems in the workplace: Key issues and a research agenda. *Psychiatry Service, 58*, 1262–1264.

Nieuwenhuijsen, K., Verbeek, J. H. A. M., De Boer, A. G. E. M., Blonk, R. W. B., & Van Dijk, F. J. H. (2004). Supervisory behaviour as a predictor of return to work in employees absent from work due to mental health problems. *Occupational and Environmental Medicine, 61*, 817–823.

Prochaska, J. O., & Di Clemente, C. C. (1982). Transtheoretical therapy: Toward a more integrative model of change. *Psychotherapy: Theory, Research, and Practice, 19*, 276–288.

Reynolds, G. S., & Lehman, W. E. (2003). Levels of substance use and willingness to use the employee assistance program. *The Journal of Behavioral Health Services & Research, 30*, 238–248.

Saks, A. M., Haccoun, R. R., & Belcourt, M. (2004). *Managing performance through training and development.* Scarborough, ON: Nelson.

Sauter, S. L., Murphy, L. R., & Hurrell, Jr., J. J. (1990). Prevention of work-related psychological disorders. *American Psychologist, 45*, 1146–1153.

Schaufeli, W. B., & Bakker, A. B. (2004). Job demands, job resources, and their relationship with burnout and engagement: A multi-sample study. *Journal of Organizational Behavior, 25*, 293–315.

Schaufeli, W. B., Salanova, M., González-Romá, V., & Bakker, A. B. (2002). The measurement of engagement and burnout: A two sample confirmatory factor analytic approach. *Journal of Happiness Studies, 3*, 71–92.

Schumm, J. A., Briggs-Phillips, M., & Hobfoll, S. E. (2006). Cumulative interpersonal traumas and social support as risk and resiliency factors in predicting PTSD and depression among inner-city women. *Journal of Traumatic Stress, 19*, 825–836.

Sonnentag, S., Kuttler, I., & Fritz, C. (2010). Job stressors, emotional exhaustion, and need for recovery: A multi-source study on the benefits of psychological detachment. *Journal of Vocational Behavior, 76*, 355–365.

Stead, R., Shanahan, M. J., & Neufeld, R. W. (2010). "I'll go to therapy, eventually": Procrastination, stress and mental health. *Personality and Individual Differences, 49*, 175–180.

Steinberg, M., & Gottlieb, B. H. (1994). The appraisal of spousal support by women facing conflicts between work and family. In B. R. Burleson, T. L. Albrecht, & I. G. Sarason (Eds.), *Communication of social support: Messages, interactions, relationships, and community.* Thousand Oaks, CA: Sage.

Swann, W. B., & Predmore, S. C. (1985). Intimates as agents of social support: Sources of consolation or despair? *Journal of Personality and Social Psychology, 49*, 1609–1617.

Tardy, C. H. (1994). Counteracting task-induced stress: Studies of instrumental and emotional support in problem-solving contexts. In B. R. Burleson, T. L. Albrecht, & I. G. Sarason (Eds.), *Communication of social support: Messages, interactions, relationships, and community* (pp. 71–87). Thousand Oaks, CA: Sage.

Tice, D. M., & Baumeister, R. F. (1997). Longitudinal study of procrastination, performance, stress, and health: The costs and benefits of dawdling. *Psychological Science, 8*, 454–458.

U.S. Department of Health and Human Services. (1999). *Mental health: A report of the surgeon general.* Rockville, MD: U.S. Department of Health and Human Services, Substance Abuse and Mental Health Services Administration, Center for Mental Health Services, National Institute of Health, National Institute of Mental Health.

U.S. Department of Labor, Bureau of Labor Statistics. (2005). *National compensation survey: Employee benefits in private industry in the United States.* Retrieved from www.bls.gov/ncs/ebs/sp/ebsm0003.pdf

Van der Doef, M., & Maes, S. (1999). The job demand-control(-support) model and psychological well-being: A review of 20 years of empirical research. *Work & Stress, 13*, 87–114.

Wells, J. D., Hobfoll, S. E., & Lavin, J. (1999). When it rains, it pours: The greater impact of resource loss compared to gain on psychological distress. *Personality and Social Psychology Bulletin, 25,* 1172–1182.

World Health Organization. (2004). *The summary report on promoting mental health: Concepts, emerging evidence, and practice.* Geneva: World Health Organization.

# HOLISTIC LEADER DEVELOPMENT: A TOOL FOR ENHANCING LEADER WELL-BEING

Cathleen Clerkin and Marian N. Ruderman

## ABSTRACT

*Today's work environment requires a new type of leader development. It is no longer enough for leaders to be qualified and knowledgeable. Leaders must be focused, adaptable, and resilient in order to be effective amid the increasingly distracting and chaotic organizational world. We argue that current methods of leader development need to evolve to encompass leader well-being and focus on intrapersonal competencies in order to adequately prepare leaders for today's stressful work world. We provide a holistic development framework for leaders which we believe is a better match for the intrapersonal capabilities required by leadership roles. Our approach is two-fold. First, we believe it is important to educate leaders on the potential interaction between the external sources of stress and leaders' neurophysiological and subjective well-being. Second, we believe leaders need different development experiences, ones that can help renew psychological resources. We review four categories of holistic*

The Role of Leadership in Occupational Stress
Research in Occupational Stress and Well Being, Volume 14, 161–186
Copyright © 2016 by Emerald Group Publishing Limited
All rights of reproduction in any form reserved
ISSN: 1479-3555/doi:10.1108/S1479-355520160000014007

*leadership practices — mindfulness, social connections, positive emotion inductions, and body-based practices — which can help to counter the effects of overload and exhaustion. We also discuss the future of holistic leader development and suggest directions for future research.*

**Keywords:** Holistic; neuroscience; leader development; leader; mindfulness

The world is changing rapidly and the workplace is changing along with it. Technology has changed the pace, location, and nature of work, creating an unprecedented degree of choice regarding what to focus on, as well as when and where to work. Historically, such workplace flexibility has been viewed positively because it allows for increased autonomy and ownership; however, the digital-era wave of options has created a double-edged sword for leaders. Along with the ability to work flexible hours has come the expectation to work beyond the traditional work week. The ability to "log on" from remote locations has created the pressure for leaders to never go offline (Deal, 2013). Access to instant information has led to the perceived need to multitask and to get things done more rapidly. Moreover, leaders today must respond to a high level of ambiguity, complexity, and uncertainty shaped by a global marketplace and economic upheavals (Darling, 2012). Unsurprisingly, these changes in workplace contexts have also come with increased reports of negative well-being. In fact, a recent study by the American Psychological Association (2015) estimates that 60% of Americans view work as a somewhat or very significant source of stress.

However, despite the growing issue of unhealthy workplace practices at the organizational level, there has been little movement in systematically cultivating well-being at the *leader development* level. We believe that this is a notable oversight, given that a number of studies have demonstrated that leaders often set the tone for their organizations. Leaders have been shown to influence the ethics of their organizational culture (Huhtala, Kangas, Lämsä, & Feldt, 2013); the way that conflict is handled in organizations (Gelfand, Leslie, Keller, & de Dreu, 2012), organizational learning and innovation (García-Morales, Jiménez-Barrionuevo, & Gutiérrez-Gutiérrez, 2012), and occupational injuries (Barling, Loughlin, & Kelloway, 2002), just to list a few examples. Given this, we believe that leaders play a key role in modeling, supporting, and sustaining healthy approaches to coping with an increasingly potentially unhealthy work environment.

We believe that leader development is an appropriate and critical venue for cultivating leader well-being practices. Leader development can be defined as the "expansion of a person's capacity to be effective in leadership roles and processes" (McCauley, Van Veslor, & Ruderman, 2010, p. 2).[1] Leader development can be a means of reducing the negative effects of job stresses associated with leadership positions (Boyatzis, Smith, & Blaize, 2006), and can help leaders better sustain themselves in the contemporary world (Kelloway & Barling, 2010).

This chapter explores a perspective on leader development which can help executives and managers better respond to the stresses of the current leadership environment, which can in turn help nurture more healthy practices in the workplace at large. In particular, we build on the idea that a fundamental aspect of being a leader is understanding *intrapersonal* competencies. This differs from more traditional HR approaches to leader development which focuses primarily on gaining skills and behaviors. We hone in on intrapersonal competencies because we believe they are most vital to leveraging leader development as a means of enhancing well-being, focus, adaptability, and resilience in the modern world.

Day (2000) argues that there are three types of intrapersonal competencies related to leader development: *self-awareness*, *self-regulation*, and *self-motivation*. It is these intrapersonal competencies that help leaders ameliorate the impact of stressful environments in order to lead effectively. For example, leaders have a responsibility to continually put the good of the organization over their own personal needs, recognize that they are role models for the collective, prioritize problems, and figure out how to best interact with others. The constant demand for control over the self can be depleting and stressful (Baumeister, Heatherton, & Tice, 1994). Continually sustaining this requires being able to renew internal, psychological resources. A well-being-based approach to leader development emphasizes the development of the dynamic psychological resources needed for continually being able to self-regulate and focus in the face of uncertainty and competing demands (Fig. 1).

In this chapter, we argue that holistic, well-being-based leader development interventions can reduce the impact of work stress on people in leadership positions, and by proxy, improve the well-being of the workplace. Our chapter develops this holistic perspective by first looking at the impact of the environment on leaders' well-being and then moving on to discuss recommended practices for developing leaders better able to function in the

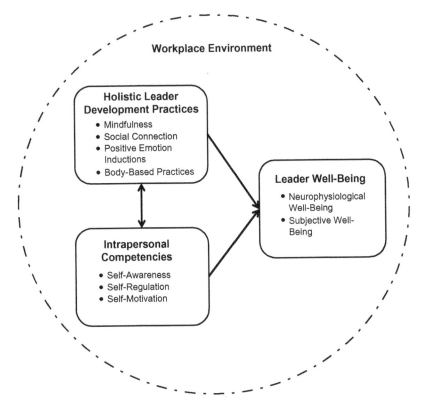

*Fig. 1.* Holistic Well-Being-Based Approach to Leader Development.

face of stress. Our approach to holistic leader development is informed by the latest findings in affective neuroscience, physiology, and positive psychology. Following Meurs and Perrewé (2011), we believe in the integration of other disciplines for understanding organization-based experiences.

## THE RELATIONSHIP BETWEEN WORK ENVIRONMENT AND LEADER WELL-BEING

Given the realities of the changes in the workplace, we believe that the development of leaders needs to focus on how to train leaders to adapt, flex, and bounce back in an ambiguous and unpredictable unknown future. The first step in the process of using leader development to enhance well-being is to examine the factors in the environment that interact with intrapersonal competences and deplete psychological resources. We have already mentioned some of the external environmental factors: long work hours, unrealistic expectations, distracting technology, competing priorities, and volatile economies and work environments. Most leaders are aware of these types of external challenges and can fairly readily describe these external sources of interference.

However, most leaders are not fully aware of how these factors influence their internal, physical, and psychological functioning. The impact of these factors on self-regulation and other intrapersonal competencies is significant but not well understood. In the following sections, we provide some examples of how external factors interact with internal processes to increase or decrease leaders' well-being. Recognition of these dynamics is a starting place for a holistic perspective on leader development. For the sake of simplicity, we focus on two broad areas of scientific interest – neurophysiological well-being and subjective well-being, along with examples of how each can impact leaders' overall ability to lead organizations.

### *Leaders' Neurophysiological Well-Being*

We use the term *neurophysiological well-being* to encompass the relative functioning and health of the physical, chemical, and neurological aspects of leaders' brains and bodies. All human behavior and actions are greatly influenced by the basic network of interconnected neurons in the brain and nervous system. Leaders are no exception. Therefore, we believe that increased understanding and awareness of neurophysiological health can help leaders better understand their own and others' bodies and behaviors, and in turn, learn more adaptive responses in stressful and volatile situations.

Research demonstrates that neurophysiological health can impact how individuals process and remember information, their decision-making ability, and their interpersonal interactions – aspects vital to leadership performance. As the pace and complexity of dilemmas increase in the future, leaders' neurophysiological fitness will matter more than ever. Yet, the very resources that keep leaders mentally recharged and healthy – e.g., adequate sleep, healthy nutrition, exercise, meditative time, down time, time with family and friends, focused time, and play time (Siegel, 2012) – are most likely to be cast aside in the face of those dilemmas. All of these activities have been shown to be important to promoting neurophysiological health, and we believe all of them should be incorporated into the fabric of leader development programs. Below are two examples of how knowledge about neurophysiological health can inform and be incorporated into leader development.

*The Impact of Sleep Deprivation on Leadership*
Sleep plays a vital role in learning, memory, and focus; during sleep, neural networks in the brain encode, process, and integrate the day's experiences with previously stored information in ways that make it available for future use (Ellenbogen, Payne, & Stickgold, 2006). Conversely, sleep deprivation can lead to decreased short-term and long-term memory, diminished focus, and slower responses, making it difficult to make decisions and to learn from mistakes (Walker, Stickgold, Alsop, Gaab, & Schlaug, 2005). Sleep deprivation also impairs mood regulation, often leading to anxiety and hostility (Connolly, Ruderman, & Leslie, 2013). Over time, sleep deprivation damages physical wellness, leading to consequences that include higher risks of accidents, diabetes, heart disease, and hypertension (King et al., 2008; Knutson, Ryden, Mander, & Van Cauter, 2006; Williamson & Feyer, 2000).

One of the primary tasks of leaders is to make important decisions — often while under pressure and with serious consequences. Lack of sleep could cause lapses in judgment or memory and lead to detrimental errors. Indeed, one hospital study found that approximately 25% of ICU errors made by first year medical interns could be accounted for by sleep deprivation caused by long work hours (Lockley et al., 2004). Another study found that individuals who stayed awake for 24 hours straight had cognitive and motor impairment similar to individuals with a blood alcohol level of 0.10 (Williamson & Feyer, 2000). Lack of mood and emotion regulation caused by sleep deprivation could also make it hard for leaders to communicate effectively and engage in the interpersonal processes necessary for successful leadership (Connolly et al., 2013). Long-term sleep deprivation is likely to lead to increased sick days, medical bills, and leaves of absence.

Helping leaders gain self-awareness on the importance of sleep is a crucial step to ameliorate the negative effects the current 24/7 work culture has not only on leaders' health, but also on sustainable organizational success. Increased awareness about sleep health is particularly important in an era of global leadership in which leaders might be required to attend conference calls in the middle of the night or fly between offices on the weekend. We suggest future leader development programs explain the importance of sleep and provide information on good sleep hygiene.

*The Impact of Threat Responses on Leadership*
A second way that leaders' neurophysiology can affect leadership effectiveness is via the neurochemical reactions to threats in the work environment.
When individuals are confronted with external stressors, neurochemicals
are released in the amygdala and hypothalamus areas of the brain, which
sends signals to the adrenal glands to pump epinephrine (i.e., adrenaline)
into the bloodstream, causing increased heart rate, blood pressure, alert-
ness, and sensory acuity. After the initial wave of adrenaline crashes,
follow-up hormones are released, including cortisol (the hormone associated with stress). Cortisol levels stay elevated until after the external situation passes, at which point the parasympathetic nervous system calms the
body and recalibrates hormone and transmitter levels.

This complicated chemical reaction — aka the "fight, flight, freeze"
response — evolved as a short-term, emergency response to help humans
survive physically threatening situations (Sapolsky, 2004). However, this
response has become increasingly maladaptive in a modern leadership
environment where external threats and stressors are more likely to be
social than life endangering, and more likely to be chronic than fleeting.
Yet, our automatic chemical responses do not differentiate between
physical or psychological threats. Today's leaders find themselves facing
sustained heightened chemical stress levels which can damage neuron
dendrites, and prevent new neurons from forming, leading to faulty communication between brain cells (Chetty et al., 2014; Pavlides, Nivón, &
McEwen, 2002). These physiological changes in turn damages information
flow in the brain, leading to decreased memory, learning, decision-making,
problem-solving, and focus (Pavlides et al., 2002; Sapolsky, 2004). Chronic
stress is also linked to a number of psychological and physical ailments,
including heart disease, high blood pressure, diabetes, depression, anxiety,
mood disorders, and lowered immune system functioning (Carlson, 2004;
Chetty et al., 2014).

As with sleep deprivation, the impact of chronic stress on leadership
ability is clear and profound. Leaders are responsible for remembering a
myriad of information, making challenging decisions, and staying calm and
focused, all while under a great deal of pressure. Thus, humans' default
neurochemical responses essentially create a handicap for leaders in the
contemporary world. We believe that an important part of the leader development process is to help leaders understand how internal processes such
as threat reactions affect leadership ability, and to provide steps and techniques in aid of stress management. An increasing amount of research

suggests that with training and practice, people can be taught to change their automatic stress responses (addressed further later in this chapter).

## Leaders' Subjective Well-Being

Subjective well-being can be defined as an individual's cognitive and emotional evaluation of one's life (Diener, Oishi, & Lucas, 2003). The study of subjective well-being examines how people's emotional reactions, moods, thoughts, and judgments about events in their life shape their overall life satisfaction and well-being. Leaders' subjective well-being is a critical factor in how they handle stressful workplace environments. According to Richard Lazarus' theory of stress, stress is the combined result of external environmental stressors coupled with individuals' subjective interpretation of the stressors (Lazarus, 1993). As such, stress can be thought of as what happens when people do not feel that they have adequate resources to cope with external demands (Lazarus, 1966).

Subjective well-being has been shown to be related to organizational well-being, including higher employee retention and performance (Page & Vella-Brodrick, 2009). Similarly, positive workplace cultures, such as high performance work systems, can enhance subjective well-being (Fan et al., 2014). We believe that leaders can be taught to increase their subjective well-being through boosting intrapersonal competencies, allowing leaders to feel that they have more internal resources to help them cope with external demands. Holistic development can help individuals reappraise their initial cognitive and emotional reactions and reinterpret events in ways that provide more subjective well-being. Additionally, given that research shows that readiness for self-improvement is a strong predictor of subjective well-being in the workplace (Zawadzka & Szabowska-Walaszczyk, 2014), leader development may be a particularly appropriate way to instill subjective well-being strategies, because leaders attend leader development with the goal of self-improvement. One example of how individuals' cognitive and emotional evaluations of events can impact leader performance is via rumination.

### The Impact of Rumination on Leadership

Rumination is the act of repetitively and passively thinking about the causes, symptoms, and effects of one's problems and/or negative feelings (Nolen-Hoeksema & Morrow, 1991). People who ruminate get caught in negative thought spirals, replaying negative events in their lives over and over. According to a review by Nolen-Hoeksema and colleagues, individuals generally report ruminating as a means of problem-solving; yet rumination inherently focuses on errors, rather than solutions, and has been related to poor problem-solving ability (Nolen-Hoeksema, Wisco, & Lyubomirsky, 2008). Rumination has also been linked to a number of other negative psychological and performance outcomes, including avoidance, poor attention, depression, anxiety, self-sabotage, low confidence, and decreased social networks and support systems (Nolen-Hoeksema et al., 2008).

Given that rumination has been shown to decrease cognitive functioning such as attention and problem-solving, it is likely to be particularly harmful to leaders' effectiveness in today's fast paced and high-pressure work environment. Indeed, previous research has established a link between rumination and workplace stress (Berset, Elfering, Lüthy, Lüthi, & Semmer, 2011). Moreover, high-performing leaders with demanding workloads might be particularly susceptible to ruminating (Syrek & Antoni, 2014). Leaders who ruminate could lose the support of their followers − which in turn would likely cause more rumination. Research has shown that emotions are contagious and that followers often look to leaders to understand how to respond in stressful and trying situations (Barsade, 2002). Leaders who demonstrate negative affect and who ruminate over past failures are likely to spread these feelings and responses throughout their team − leading to a group of people who lack the direction and motivation to change negative situations into positive ones.

Importantly, people can be taught to stop ruminating (Nolen-Hoeksema et al., 2008). Thus, leader development programs could train individuals to recognize ruminative patterns and redirect them. This type of development could help leaders not only self-regulate better, but also better manage the emotions of others. Research shows that simple methods such as redirecting one's focus something positive and attention consuming can distract ruminative thoughts and break down negativity cycles (Nolen-Hoeksema et al., 2008). However, these methods take time and discipline to perfect, and little research has been done to establish how leader development programs might best incorporate such practices. In the next section, we take a closer look at self-modification techniques and how such concepts might be introduced into the field of leader development.

## HOLISTIC LEADER DEVELOPMENT PRACTICES

Traditional approaches to leader development focus on the *what* of leader behaviors. In contrast, our holistic approach to leader development focuses on the *how* of leadership in terms of consciously engaging in self-modification in order to boost well-being and resilience. For leaders to succeed today, they need to improve skills in observing, modifying, and regulating various mental processes. The goal of holistic leader development is to increase leaders' abilities to fine tune their inner processes, allowing leaders to better exercise control over the self.

There are a number of holistic tools, techniques, and principles which can help leaders build their intrapersonal capabilities. In this section, we offer four examples of such practices: (1) mindfulness practices, (2) social connections, (3) positive emotion inductions, and (4) body-based practices. Although the supportive evidence for each of these techniques varies, each of them has some promise for helping individuals become more aware, proactive, and deliberate regarding their thoughts, emotions, actions, and behaviors. Most of the evidence for these practices comes from disciplines other than leader development, and future research is needed to integrate them into the field. Thus, we offer the following sections to illustrate the potential of what holistic leader development might be like, rather than to review current leader development programs. See Table 1 for a summary of

*Table 1.* Holistic Leader Development Methods.

| Holistic Leader Development Practices | Forms, Tools, and Applications | General Performance and Well-Being Outcomes |
|---|---|---|
| Mindfulness | Concentrative techniques, awareness-based techniques, guided techniques, MBSR programs, mindful journaling, mindful eating, and metaphor techniques. | Increased attention, memory, emotion regulation, psychological well-being, immune function, and empathy. Decreased bias, stress, and pain, illness. |
| Social connection | High-quality connections, reciprocity rings, networking, career coaching, mentors, and social events. | Increased memory, immune system, and job satisfaction. Decreased stress, cognitive decline, and risky behavior. |
| Positive emotion inductions | Loving-kindness practices, gratitude journaling, gratitude contemplation, gratitude letters, gratitude visits, emotional and facial training and feedback. | Increased well-being, creativity, life and job satisfaction, executive brain functioning, resilience, and interpersonal savvy. Decreased depression. |
| Body-based practices | Yoga, Tai Chi, cardiovascular activity, nature walks, body scans, Feldenkrais, and "playing it out." | Increased physical health, mood, and self-esteem. Decreased stress, anxiety, and depression. |

these practices, common tools, and applications, and established performance and wellness outcomes.

## Mindfulness Practices

There are many definitions of mindfulness, but perhaps the best known in the contemporary Western world is Kabat-Zinn's definition of "paying attention, in a particular way, on purpose" with a non-judgmental attitude (1994, p. 4). Mindfulness can be thought of as a present-centered awareness in which thoughts and feelings are observed as products of the mind rather than as factual realities. Mindfulness heightens awareness of how thoughts and emotions impact behaviors, sharpening one's sense of what is happening in the moment rather than letting anxieties, worries, and distractions overpower the experience of the here and now (Kabat-Zinn, 1994). There are a number of tools and methods that can be used to facilitate mindfulness, many of which involve some form of meditation; common methods include concentrative techniques, awareness-based techniques, guided techniques, mindful journaling, and metaphor techniques.

### Performance and Well-Being Outcomes

The literature on mindfulness is fairly well-established, and much of the latest research comes from social cognitive psychology and neuroscience. Cognitively, there is evidence that mindfulness training can enhance attentional control (Jha, Krompinger, & Baime, 2007), working memory and emotion regulation (Bishop et al., 2004), psychological well-being (Brown & Ryan, 2003), and limit biases (Hafenbrack, Kinias, & Barsade, 2014). Theory suggests that mindfulness improves cognitive processes by providing practice in the skill of intercepting automatic reactions and shifting thoughts (Baer, 2003). This is sometimes referred to as "decentering" – standing back and witnessing thoughts and feelings instead of being immersed and caught up in them (Baer, 2003). This is especially important in the face of stressful situations or negative emotional states, which might evoke suboptimal automatic behaviors. Mindful emotion regulation also facilitates improved interpersonal relationships, via increased capacity for compassion and empathy (Sedlmeier et al., 2012).

Research has also shown that mindfulness can impact neurophysiological health. Mindfulness practices have been associated with increased cortical thickness, suggesting that mindfulness can change the physiology of the brain (Kerr, Sacchet, Lazar, Jones, & Moore, 2013; Lazar et al., 2005).

There is also evidence that mindfulness can reduce cortisol levels (Carlson, Campbell, Garland, & Grossman, 2007) and enhance immune function (Davidson et al., 2003). Correspondingly, mindfulness breathing meditation has been linked to decreased illness and depressive symptoms and increased stress management (Fredrickson, Cohn, Coffey, Pek, & Finkel, 2008; Kabat-Zinn, 1991; Sapolsky, 2004).

However, it should be noted that recent research has begun to explore the possible negative impacts of mindfulness. For example, research from the University of San Diego has shown that mindfulness experiences can result in vulnerability to false memories (Wilson, Mickes, Stolarz-Fantino, Evrard, & Fantino, 2015). Mindfulness exercises are intended to demonstrate that thoughts are not facts. In doing so, it may inhibit some of the processes that actually help distinguish true from false memories. Further research needs to evaluate the parameters of such side effects relative to the benefits.

*Leader Applications and Future Directions*
While mindfulness has been around for over two millennia (mostly within Eastern religious and spiritual practices), it is only recently that these techniques have been applied into Western efforts to facilitate human potential. Recent years have seen a large influx of mindfulness interventions in the workplace (Hyland, Lee, & Mills, 2015). Mindfulness programs, especially Mindfulness-Based Stress Reduction programs, have become particularly popular within healthcare facilities and have been proven to help with coping with pain, anxiety, and depression (Kabat-Zinn, 1991). Recently, a number of organizations and education systems have also started to incorporate mindfulness into their institutions in order to encourage focus, memory, lower stress, and facilitate learning (Gelles, 2012).

While less effort has been made to incorporate mindfulness into leader development programs specifically, there is reason to believe that this is a promising avenue for future research and application (Ruderman & Clerkin, 2015). Mindfulness practices could help leaders better attend to the world through increasing focus and decision-making, and by acting with more considered, unbiased responses. By increasing awareness of the present, mindfulness practices open up the possibility of responding intentionally rather than reactively to modern organizational challenges. In a systematic review of the literature, Bishop et al. (2004) propose that the central mechanism underlying meditative techniques is metacognition, or insight into one's own thinking process. Developing leaders to be able to recognize their own internal workings could go a long way to helping leaders navigate volatile and unpredictable contexts and develop the empathy and emotional balance needed for effective leadership.

## Social Connection

Humans are intrinsically social beings and development and growth occurs in relationship with one another. A substantial body of research shows that social connection is important not only for physical survival, but also for psychological well-being and cognitive flourishing (Siegel, 2012). Socially driven constructs such as social support, social ties, networking, social integration, and teamwork have all been linked to improved performance and outcomes both within organizational contexts, and in society in general.

### Performance and Well-Being Outcomes

There is an abundance of research on the power of relationships on cognitive and neurophysiological health and well-being. For instance, longitudinal data from the Health and Retirement study showed that people with the highest levels of social integration had less cognitive decline and better memory compared to less socially active subjects (Ertel, Glymour, & Berkman, 2008). Similarly, people who were infected with the rhinovirus were less likely to develop colds if they had more types of social ties (Cohen, Doyle, Skoner, Rabin, & Gwaltney, 1997). Neurological findings support the idea that one person can affect another's emotions and well-being. For example, one study found that during stressful situations, individuals' brains become calmer (i.e., threat-related neural activation decreases) when someone holds our hand (Coan, Schaefer, & Davidson, 2006). Similarly, perceived social support can buffer against physiological stress reactions (Cohen, Janicki-Deverts, Turner, & Doyle, 2015).

The positive impacts of social relationships have been demonstrated within workplace contexts as well. A meta-analysis of 68 studies suggests that social support in the workplace can reduce strains, mitigate perceived stressors, and moderate the stressor-strain relationship in stressful workplace environments (Viswesvaran, Sanchez, & Fisher, 1999). Social support has also been shown to positively predict job satisfaction and job tenure (Harris, Winskowski, & Engdahl, 2007). Even brief social interactions have been shown to have a positive cardiovascular, neuroendocrine, and immune system effects on individuals in workplace settings (Heaphy & Dutton, 2008).

On the flip side, the presence of negative relationships and social connections can be a detriment to health, well-being and life satisfaction. Studies show that stressful and unpleasant interpersonal relationships are related to increased heart rate, and blood pressure, risky behavior and unhealthy life choices such as drinking, smoking, unhealthy eating, and non-compliance to medical regimens (see Umberson & Montez, 2010 for a review). Negative workplace relationships also have a huge impact on people's lives. Abusive and bullying interactions from peers and supervisors can damage employee health and well-being, leading to increased medical leave, work dissatisfaction, quitting, and in rare cases, even suicide (Quigg, 2015).

*Leader Applications and Future Directions*
While social connections have always been a feature of the workplace, an increasing amount of research is beginning to focus on the social aspects of work in a more deliberate, structured, and facilitated way. For instance, Baker and Dutton (2007) identify two primary classes of social practices that can create and sustain social capital in the workplace: High-Quality Connections (HQCs) and reciprocity. HQCs are connections between people characterized by mutuality, positive regard, and vitality. They stand out as different from low quality connections because they have a positive and lasting impact on people through heightened positive emotions and enhanced physiological functioning (Dutton, 2014). Reciprocity has to do with the exchange of resources between people in organizations. Successful reciprocity in organizations reflects individuals' willingness to give to others.

The deliberate cultivation of positive social connections has the potential to be a powerful tool for leaders. Employees tend to look to supervisors for guidance and feedback, and therefore social connections with supervisors can have the ability to shape employees' experience of the workplace. Research shows that social exchanges between leaders and followers are predictive of a number of outcomes, including followers' performance, affective commitment to the organization, and citizenship behavior (Wayne, Shore, & Liden, 1997). As organizations adapt to constant change, leaders must create and use social capital. Strong relationships can provide resilience for individuals and groups during times of stress.

Social connections are already often one of the positive side effects of leader development programs. However, future leader development initiatives should be more deliberate and explicitly teach, facilitate, and provide opportunities to practice reciprocity and high-quality connections. For instance, Baker has developed reciprocity rings as way to teach leaders about reciprocity and for organizations to bring principles of reciprocity into their systems (humaxnetworks.com). Similarly, Dutton proposes that leaders can be taught to purposefully foster HCQs through respectful engagements, task enabling, trusting, and playing (Dutton, 2014). Moreover, skills such as career mentoring and coaching could be taught to leaders through formal mentoring and coaching training and alumni partnerships, since these skills predict follower job satisfaction and job tenure (Harris et al., 2007).

## Positive Emotion Inductions

A wealth of research in the fields of positive psychology and the psychology of emotions has shown the benefits of positive emotions. Fredrickson's broaden and build theory is often used to explain the mechanism linking positive emotions to various positive outcomes (2001). This theory suggests that during stressful times, negative emotions arise as a means of narrowing thought to allow for focusing on a specific problem. However, during safe times, positive emotions help us promote social bonds, creative thinking, and other ways of broadening our thinking and building our resources. Recent research has explored how positive emotions may be invoked or induced in order to cultivate these natural benefits.

### Performance and Well-Being Outcomes
Positive emotions have been linked to increased well-being, creativity, life satisfaction, executive brain functioning, and decreased worrying and depression (Fredrickson, 2009; Wood, Froh, & Geraghty, 2010). There is also a link between positive emotions and resilience. Resilient people tend to have higher emotion regulation and are more likely to use positive emotions to bounce back from stressful encounters (Fredrickson, 2009). Positive emotions have even been shown to precede and predict several different measures of success, including income, performance, and health, leading researchers to believe that positivity may be the catalyst to desirable characteristics, behaviors, and resources (Lyubomirsky, King, & Diener, 2005).

Within organizational contexts, positivity has been shown to be related to "upward spirals" − broadening resources and thought processes (Fredrickson, 2003). For example, individuals who were randomly assigned to practice loving-kindness meditation increased their daily experiences of positive emotions, which in turn increased their personal resources in the workplace (Fredrickson et al., 2008). Another study found that MBA students who reported more positive emotions performed more accurately and thoughtfully on a decision-making task, and demonstrated more interpersonal savvy (Fredrickson, 2003). Positive emotions such as hope and optimism have been linked to increased job satisfaction, work happiness, and organizational commitment (Youssef & Luthans, 2007); while a growing body of research suggests that gratitude in particular, can cultivate well-being in organizations (Wood et al., 2010).

*Leader Applications and Future Directions*
As with social connections, leaders play a large role in the emotional state of their organizations. Research has shown that leaders' positive emotional expressions can influence the mood states of their followers, and that both leaders and followers' emotional expressions influence ratings of leader effectiveness (Bono, Foldes, Vinson, & Muros, 2007). In a study in the IT sector, Arakawa and Greenberg (2007) found that positive leadership was correlated with employee engagement and performance, and manager optimism predicted project performance. This suggests that for leaders, not only can positive emotions impact their own well-being and performance but also that of their followers.

We believe that positivity inductions are ideal for incorporating into leader development practices. The research on inducting emotions in organizational contexts suggests that gratitude interventions might be particularly helpful. Gratitude induction approaches that could be added to leader development programs include gratitude journaling, contemplative approaches, and behavioral approaches such as writing letters of gratitude or conducting gratitude visits (Wood et al., 2010). Similarly, leaders could be instructed in how to share positive emotions and positive facial expressions in order to boost team morale. Loving-kindness practices could be introduced to help leaders connect with their own positivity. These simple tools could help leaders create upward spirals once they return to their places of work, and could have widespread benefits to their organizations.

*Body-Based Practices*

The final family of practices we review in this chapter involves physical movement and body-awareness. For centuries, the mind-body connection has been recognized by a variety of techniques such as Tai Chi, yoga, body-oriented psychotherapy, and Feldenkrais (Mehling et al., 2011). What these different physical approaches have in common is that they are designed to increase body-awareness through understanding and integrating the mind and body in order to respond to the environment more deliberately. With the cumulative changes in the environment, understanding the body as a means of sensing what is going on in the external world is an important capability.

*Performance and Well-Being Outcomes*
The benefits of physical movement and body-based practices are well known and include improved well-being, energy, and focus. In one study, four months of yoga was found to significantly improve psychological and physiological stress, mood, blood pressure, and heart rate as much as cognitive behavior therapy (Granath, Ingvarsson, von Thiele, & Lundberg, 2006). Similarly, a recent meta-analysis suggests that Tai Chi is positively related psychological well-being and self-esteem, and negatively related to stress, anxiety, depression, and mood disturbance (Wang et al., 2010). While many researchers and practitioners espouse the importance of body-based practices that hone in on the mind-body connection, even simple physical activity also has neurological benefits, promoting brain development and neuron growth (Medina, 2008). A review of the literature shows that different forms of exercise moderate cognitive decline in aging (Bherer, Erickson, & Liu-Ambrose, 2013).

A variety of forms of yoga, Tai Chi, and other mind-body connection practices are now being incorporated into organizations as a way for a high-stressed workforce to gain re-centering (Gelles, 2012). Mindful yoga has been increasingly used in organizational settings and is included in mindfulness-based stress reduction courses. One study suggests that workplace Tai Chi programs can improve musculoskeletal fitness and psychological well-being among computer users (Tamim et al., 2009). Other studies have shown that even brief, low impact physical activity interventions in the workplace can improve employees' physical health (Yancey et al., 2004).

*Leader Applications and Future Directions*
Most of the research on physical wellness is not tied directly to leadership. However, given the evidence that activity and cognition are related, the potential for physical movement to improve leadership ability exists. In particular, research demonstrating that physical movement and mind-body practices can reduce stress and increase memory and cognitive performance suggests that physical approaches are useful for a leadership population. In one of the few examinations of exercise in a leadership population, McDowell-Larsen argues that leaders' brain health can be enhanced through exercise, sleep, and diet (McDowell-Larsen, 2012).

In addition to such mind-body wellness practices as mentioned above, we also see body-based practices as a way to help leaders physically deal with stress. As we previously described, the body responds to threat automatically – secreting hormones and increasing heart rates to prepare for fight-flight-freeze responses. Since none of these responses are acceptable in a business environment, leaders can end up with an overdose of cortisol in their systems after years of stressful work-life. According to Evans (2015), one way that leaders can reinstate equilibrium is to "play it out" – participate in short bursts of intense movement to use up extra cortisol. This practice of physically dealing with energy and stress can take multiple forms, such as running up the stairs in an office building, using a punching bag or jumping rope. We believe that training leaders to physically regulate their stress reaction has the potential to have a great impact.

The application for incorporating body-based practices into leader development is fairly straight forward. Body-based techniques allow leaders to increase their mind-body connection and provide a way to redirect visceral reactions to difficult situations. Additionally, given that some research suggests that fitness-based programs are hard to integrate into the workplace (Marshall, 2004), leaders can also play important roles in modeling physical well-being in their organizations. While there is a long history of using various body-based practices in sports training and meditative traditions, these practices have been fairly absent from leader development programs. A lot of research needs to be done on which practices are most related to leadership abilities, and how to best implement the practices into leader development. For a meaningful shift to occur, development programs should explore how to create physical habits so that the body can more easily recover from stress and threatening issues can be reevaluated and responded to from a position of greater clarity.

*Future Directions: Technology-Based Holistic Leader Development*

In addition to the holistic practices described above, we also believe that new technological advancements can provide opportunities for holistic leader development. Technology is improving at an exponential rate, and many new technological innovations have clear and direct implications for health, well-being, and behavioral modification. However, to date, most of the technological offerings in this area seem to lack the dexterity and nuance needed to provide meaningful leader development. Never the less, we provide a brief discussion of technology-based tools here, as we believe they hold potential for the near future of leader development.

*Brain Training*

Brain training describes the attempt to enhance cognitive abilities via various types of games and mental activities – e.g., online games, crossword puzzles, Sudoku, or ken-ken. There is currently a growing industry selling computer program "brain-teasers" which claim to enhance cognitive functions such as memory, problem-solving, attention, processing speed, and navigation. However, these claims are typically based on previous, separately conducted research establishing links between cognitive activity and desired outcomes.

While there is a lot of hype and promise about brain training, the scientific evidence is mixed and preliminary. Brain-training methods are based largely on studies of brain imaging and analysis, and stem from early findings demonstrating that training may have a cognitive and physical impact on the brain (e.g., see Colom et al., 2012; Maguire et al., 2000). These and other similar studies demonstrated that the structure and density of the brain can change in response to practice at specific tasks. Based on such evidence, a number of groups have attempted to create automated brain-training programs designed to promote the type of cognitive stimulation that is required to boost cognitive ability and increase cortical thickness. However, thus far, the attempts to codify and quantify such growth have not been well validated by research. In a 2014 letter, The Stanford Center for Longevity and the Max Planck Institute for Human Development in Berlin released a statement questioning the claims that these online training programs can reduce or reverse cognitive decline associated with aging. Moreover, a comprehensive analysis by the BBC and Cambridge University of over 11,000 subjects found that while individuals who played commercialized brain-training games were more proficient on the games themselves, there were no transfer effects to general cognitive abilities (Owen et al., 2010).

*Body-Based Feedback Devices*

Another group of technological tools that could be used for leader development are body-based feedback devices. For instance, biofeedback devices use technology to access physiological health and provide feedback to the individual about the current physical state of their body. A common example is the "smart" watch, which provides the wearer with information about their heart rate and movement. Other examples include Fitbits, chest-strap heart monitors, wireless electroencephalogram caps, etc. Because many such devices are worn, they are often referred to as "wearables." However, biofeedback technology can also take on non-wearable forms, such as smartphone camera heart rate monitors, or handheld devices that calculate skin conductivity. Additionally, a growing number of body-based feedback devices provide "affective computing" or emotional feedback, such as programs which analyze facial expressions or voice tone.

Many biofeedback devices have originated from the healthcare sector, and there is substantial evidence that medical grade biofeedback technologies are fairly accurate ways to assess physiological wellness. However, as cheaper and lower grade options flood the market — often with designs originating from marketing campaigns rather than science or medicine — there has been little quality control, and the accuracy of most remain questionable (Bai et al., 2016; Luxton, McCann, Bush, Mishkind, & Reger, 2011). Moreover, to date, there is even less evidence that such devices are able to help people *modify* their behavior rather than just record it. However, a few preliminary studies suggest that these technologies, coupled with training, may enhance physical recovery and stress management (Alabdulgader, 2012).

Although thus far the findings suggest that technology-based development such as brain training and feedback devices by itself may not have much impact, future research is still warranted. It may be that current limitations of technology have kept brain-training programs and feedback devices from being refined and sophisticated enough to have concrete well-being benefits, but in the future this may change. If these technology-based methods are established as viable and scientifically sound ways to build cognitive ability, physiological health, and emotional awareness, the benefits for leadership and leader development could be profound. Brain-training targets the executive functioning areas of the brain and seeks to boost capabilities such as memory, problem-solving, focus, and attention — abilities that greatly increase leadership potential and performance. Similarly, technology-based feedback devices and wearables are designed to help hone self-awareness, self-regulation, and self-motivation — the very components of intrapersonal leader development. However, more research is needed before conclusions can be made about how to best incorporate these technology-based training methods into leader development programs, if they should be included at all.

## CONCLUSION

We believe that leaders must be more aware of how their neurophysiological and cognitive processes interact with the environment, and must learn to self-regulate and modify their internal processes in order to be successful in today's world of constant change and increasing distractions.

We propose that one way to help leaders to build these capabilities is through holistic leader development programs that focus on well-being and resilience in order to develop leaders from the inside out. The importance of these holistic practices for cultivating leadership excellence is two-fold. First, these practices can help leaders become more aware, proactive, and deliberate around their thoughts, emotions, and behaviors. Second, in building these abilities, leaders will also sharpen their understanding of others' thoughts, emotions, and behaviors – skills both necessary and invaluable to leading others effectively. With improved skills for looking inward, leaders can better look outward and engage and develop others.

We believe that holistic methods, such as those introduced in this chapter can be combined in a variety of ways and joined with other channels of development to support the larger goals of a leader development initiative. In presenting these techniques to enhance leader development, we suggest a multi-modal approach, integrating these practices with traditional behavioral development. The practices for holistic leadership development we introduced in this chapter are merely examples and are not intended to be exhaustive. Nor are they necessarily completely mutually exclusive; indeed some developmental experiences may facilitate more than one practice (e.g., gratitude visits are likely to spark both positive emotions and social connections). However, they do stand in contrast to other processes and strategies which we know are ineffective – and often detrimental – in the leadership environment, such as avoidance, ignoring, self-numbing, over-working, multi-tasking, or ruminating.

Our approach to leader development is interdisciplinary, drawing from research in neuroscience, contemplative practices, positive psychology, among others, in order to integrate methods and results that have been shown to improve human ability and potential. We believe that such integrated and interdisciplinary approaches are required to bridge the gap between the competencies needed to perform behaviors and the aspects of well-being necessary to adapt to volatile organizational environments. It is important to note that we do not suggest that behavioral competencies are no longer needed, but simply that they are no longer enough to develop successful leaders in the global workplace. Given that much of the evidence provided in this chapter come from other disciplines, future research is needed to determine which of these methods are most useful to leader development and the precise impact that mindfulness, social connection, positivity, and body-based practices may have on leaders and their organizations. We invite leadership researchers and practitioners to explore these future possibilities with us.

# NOTE

1. Leader development stands in contrast to leader*ship* development, which refers to expansion of the collective's capacity to be effective (McCauley et al., 2010).

# REFERENCES

Alabdulgader, A. A. (2012). Coherence: A novel nonpharmacological modality for lowering blood pressure in hypertensive patients. *Global Advances in Health and Medicine, 1*(2), 56–64.

American Psychological Association. (2015, February 24). *Stress in America™ paying with our health.* Retrieved from http://apa.org/news/press/releases/stress/2014/stress-report.pdf

Arakawa, D., & Greenberg, M. (2007). Optimistic managers and their influence on productivity and employee engagement in a technology organisation: Implications for coaching psychologists. *International Coaching Psychology Review, 2*(1), 78–89.

Baer, R. A. (2003). Mindfulness training as a clinical intervention: A conceptual and empirical Review. *Clinical Psychology: Science and Practice, 10*(2), 125–143.

Bai, Y., Welk, G. J., Nam, Y. H., Lee, J. A., Lee, J. M., Kim, Y., … Dixon, P. M. (2016). Comparison of consumer and research monitors under semistructured settings. *Medicine and Science in Sports and Exercise, 48*(1), 151–158.

Baker, W., & Dutton, J. E. (2007). Enabling positive social capital in organizations. In J. E. Dutton & B. R. Ragins (Eds.), *Exploring positive relationships at work: Building a theoretical and research foundation. LEA's organization and management series.* Mahwah, NJ: Lawrence Erlbaum Associates Publishers.

Barling, J., Loughlin, C. A., & Kelloway, E. K. (2002). Developmental test of a model linking safety-specific transformational leadership and occupational injuries. *Journal of Applied Psychology, 87*, 488–496. doi:10.1037/0021-9010.87.3.488

Barsade, S. (2002). The ripple effect: Emotional contagion and its influence on group behavior. *Administrative Science Quarterly, 47*, 644–675.

Baumeister, R. F., Heatherton, T. F., & Tice, D. M. (1994). *Losing control: How and why people fail at self-regulation.* San Diego, CA: Academic Press.

Berset, M., Elfering, A., Lüthy, S., Lüthi, S., & Semmer, N. K. (2011). Work stressors and impaired sleep: Rumination as a mediator. *Stress and Health, 27*(2), e71–e82.

Bherer, L., Erickson, K. I., & Liu-Ambrose, T. (2013). A review of the effects of physical activity and exercise on cognitive and brain functions in older adults. *Journal of Aging Research.* doi:10.1155/2013/657508

Bishop, S. R., Lau, M., Shapiro, S., Carlson, L., Anderson, N. D., Carmody, J., … Devins, G. (2004). Mindfulness: A proposed operational definition. *Clinical Psychology: Science and Practice, 11*(3), 230–241.

Bono, J. E., Foldes, H. J., Vinson, G., & Muros, J. P. (2007). Workplace emotions: The role of supervision and leadership. *Journal of Applied Psychology, 92*(5), 1357–1367.

Boyatzis, R. E., Smith, M. L., & Blaize, N. (2006). Developing sustainable leaders through coaching and compassion. *Academy of Management Learning & Education, 5*(1), 8–24.

Brown, K. W., & Ryan, R. M. (2003). The benefits of being present: Mindfulness and its role in psychological well-being. *Journal of Personality and Social Psychology, 84*(4), 822–848.

Carlson, N. R. (2004). *Physiology of behavior* (8th ed.). New York, NY: Allyn & Bacon.

Carlson, L. E., Campbell, T. S., Garland, S. N., & Grossman, P. (2007). Associations among salivary cortisol, melatonin, catecholamines, sleep quality and stress in women with breast cancer and healthy controls. *Journal of Behavioral Medicine, 30*(1), 45–58.

Chetty, S., Friedman, A. R., Taravosh-Lahn, K., Kirby, E. D., Mirescu, C., Guo, F., ... Kaufer, D. (2014). Stress and glucocorticoids promote oligodendrogenesis in the adult hippocampus. *Molecular Psychiatry, 19*(12), 1275–1283.

Coan, J. A., Schaefer, H. S., & Davidson, R. J. (2006). Lending a hand: Social regulation of the neural response to threat. *Psychological Science, 17*(12), 1032–1039.

Cohen, S., Doyle, W. J., Skoner, D. P., Rabin, B. S., & Gwaltney, J. M. (1997). Social ties and susceptibility to the common cold. *Journal of the American Medical Association, 277*(24), 1940–1944.

Cohen, S., Janicki-Deverts, D., Turner, R. B., & Doyle, W. J. (2015). Does hugging provide stress-buffering social support? A study of susceptibility to upper respiratory infection and illness. *Psychological Science, 26*(2), 135–147.

Colom, R., Quiroga, M. Á., Solana, A. B., Burgaleta, M., Roman, F. J., Privado, J., ... Karama, S. (2012). Structural changes after videogame practice related to a brain network associated with intelligence. *Intelligence, 40*(5), 479–489.

Connolly, C., Ruderman, M., & Leslie, J. B. (2013). *Sleep well, lead well how better sleep can improve leadership, boost productivity, and spark innovation.* White paper. Center for Creative Leadership, Greensboro, NC.

Darling, J. (2012). Global leadership: How an emerging construct is informed by complex systems theory. In J. D. Barbour, G. J. Burgess, L. L. Falkman, & R. M. McManus (Eds.), *Leading in complex worlds.* San Francisco, CA: Jossey-Bass.

Davidson, R. J., Kabat-Zinn, J., Schumacher, J., Rosenkrantz, M., Muller, D., Santorelli, S., ... Sheridan, J. (2003). Alterations in brain and immune function produced by mindfulness meditation. *Psychosomatic Medicine, 65*(4), 564–570.

Day, D. V. (2000). Leadership development: A review in context. *Leadership Quarterly, 11*, 581–613.

Deal, J. (2013). *Always on, never done: Don't blame the smartphone.* White paper. Center for Creative Leadership, Greensboro, NC.

Diener, E., Oishi, S., & Lucas, R. E. (2003). Personality, culture, and subjective well-being: Emotional and cognitive evaluations of life. *Annual Review of Psychology, 54*(1), 403–425.

Dutton, J. (2014). *How to be a positive leader through building high quality connections [PowerPoint slides].* Ann Arbor, MI: Center for Positive Organizations.

Ellenbogen, J. M., Payne, J. D., & Stickgold, R. (2006). The role of sleep in declarative memory consolidation: Passive, permissive, active or none? *Current Opinion in Neurobiology, 16*(6), 716–722.

Ertel, K. A., Glymour, M. M., & Berkman, L. F. (2008). Effects of social integration on preserving memory function in a nationally representative US elderly population. *American Journal of Public Health, 98*(7), 1215–1220.

Evans, J. C. (2015). *The resiliency rEvolution: Your stress solution for life 60 seconds at a time.* Minneapolis, MN: Wise Ink Creative Publishing.

Fan, D., Cui, L., Zhang, M. M., Zhu, C. J., Härtel, C. J., & Nyland, C. (2014). Influence of high performance work systems on employee subjective well-being and job burnout: Empirical evidence from the Chinese healthcare sector. *The International Journal of Human Resource Management, 25*(7), 931–950. doi:10.1080/09585192.2014.876740

Fredrickson, B. (2001). The role of positive emotions in positive psychology – The broaden-and-build theory of positive emotions. *American Psychologist, 56,* 218–226.

Fredrickson, B. (2009). *Positivity.* New York, NY: Three Rivers Press-Crown Publishing Group–Random House.

Fredrickson, B. L. (2003). Positive emotions and upward spirals in organizations. In K. M. Cameron, J. E. Dutton, & R. E. Quinn (Eds.), *Positive organizational scholarship* (pp. 163–175). San Francisco, CA: Berrett-Koehler.

Fredrickson, B. L., Cohn, M. A., Coffey, K. A., Pek, J., & Finkel, S. M. (2008). Open hearts build lives: Positive emotions, induced through loving-kindness meditation, build consequential personal resources. *Journal of Personality and Social Psychology, 95,* 1045–1062.

García-Morales, V. J., Jiménez-Barrionuevo, M. M., & Gutiérrez-Gutiérrez, L. (2012). Transformational leadership influence on organizational performance through organizational learning and innovation. *Journal of Business Research, 65*(7), 1040–1050.

Gelfand, M. J., Leslie, L. M., Keller, K., & de Dreu, C. (2012). Conflict cultures in organizations: How leaders shape conflict cultures and their organizational-level consequences. *Journal of Applied Psychology, 97*(6), 1131–1147. doi:10.1037/a0029993

Gelles, D. (2012). The mind business. *Financial Times,* August. Retrieved from http://www.ft.com/cms/s/2/d9cb7940-ebea-11e1-985a-00144feab49a.html

Granath, J., Ingvarsson, S., von Thiele, U., & Lundberg, U. (2006). Stress management: A randomized study of cognitive behavioural therapy and yoga. *Cognitive Behaviour Therapy, 35*(1), 3–10.

Hafenbrack, A. C., Kinias, Z., & Barsade, S. G. (2014). Debiasing the mind through meditation mindfulness and the sunk-cost bias. *Psychological Science, 25*(2), 369–376.

Harris, J. I., Winskowski, A. M., & Engdahl, B. E. (2007). Types of workplace social support in the prediction of job satisfaction. *The Career Development Quarterly, 56*(2), 150–156.

Heaphy, E. D., & Dutton, J. E. (2008). Positive social interactions and the human body at work: Linking organizations and physiology. *Academy of Management Review, 33*(1), 137–162.

Huhtala, M., Kangas, M., Lämsä, A., & Feldt, T. (2013). Ethical managers in ethical organisations? The leadership-culture connection among Finnish managers. *Leadership & Organization Development Journal, 34*(3), 250–270. doi:10.1108/01437731311326684

Hyland, P. K., Lee, R. A., & Mills, M. J. (2015). Mindfulness at work: A new approach to improving individual and organizational performance. *Industrial and Organizational Psychology, 8*(04), 576–602.

Jha, A. P., Krompinger, J., & Baime, M. J. (2007). Mindfulness training modifies subsystems of attention. *Cognitive, Affective, & Behavioral Neuroscience, 7*(2), 109–119.

Kabat-Zinn, J. (1991). *Full catastrophe living: The program of the stress reduction clinic at the University of Massachusetts Medical Center.* New York, NY: Dell.

Kabat-Zinn, J. (1994). *Wherever you go, there you are: Mindfulness meditation in everyday life.* New York, NY: Hyperion.

Kelloway, E. K., & Barling, J. (2010). Leadership development as an intervention in occupational health psychology. *Work & Stress, 24*(5), 260–279.

Kerr, C. E., Sacchet, M. D., Lazar, S. W., Jones, S. R., & Moore, C. I. (2013). Mindfulness starts with the body: Somatosensory attention and top-down modulation of cortical alpha rhythms in mindfulness meditation. *Frontiers in Human Neuroscience, 7*(12), 1–15.

King, C. R., Knutson, K. L., Rathouz, P. J., Sidney, S., Liu, K., & Lauderdale, D. S. (2008). Short sleep duration and incident coronary artery calcification. *Journal of the American Medical Association, 300*(24), 2859–2866.

Knutson, K. L., Ryden, A. M., Mander, B. A., & Van Cauter, E. (2006). Role of sleep duration and quality in the risk and severity of type 2 diabetes mellitus. *Archives of Internal Medicine, 166*(16), 1768–1774. doi:10.1001/archinte.166.16.1768

Lazar, S. W., Kerr, C. E., Wasserman, R. H., Gray, J. R., Greve, D. N., Treadway, M. T., ... Fischl, B. (2005). Meditation experience is associated with increased cortical thickness. *Neuroreport, 16*(17), 1893–1897.

Lazarus, R. S. (1966). *Psychological stress and the coping process.* New York, NY: McGraw-Hill.

Lazarus, R. S. (1993). From psychological stress to the emotions: A history of changing outlooks. *Annual Review of Psychology, 44,* 1–21.

Lockley, S. W., Cronin, J. W., Evans, E. E., Cade, B. E., Lee, C. J., Landrigan, C. P., ... Czeisler, C. A. (2004). Effect of reducing interns' weekly work hours on sleep and attentional failures. *New England Journal of Medicine, 351*(18), 1829–1837.

Luxton, D. D., McCann, R. A., Bush, N. E., Mishkind, M. C., & Reger, G. M. (2011). mHealth for mental health: Integrating smartphone technology in behavioral healthcare. *Professional Psychology: Research and Practice, 42*(6), 505–512.

Lyubomirsky, S., King, L., & Diener, E. (2005). The benefits of frequent positive affect: Does happiness lead to success? *Psychological Bulletin, 131*(6), 803–855.

Maguire, E. A., Gadian, D. G., Johnsrude, I. S., Good, C. D., Ashburner, J., Frackowiak, R. S., & Frith, C. D. (2000). Navigation-related structural change in the hippocampi of taxi drivers. *Proceedings of the National Academy of Sciences, 97*(8), 4398–4403.

Marshall, A. L. (2004). Challenges and opportunities for promoting physical activity in the workplace. *Journal of Science and Medicine in Sport, 7*(1), 60–66.

McCauley, C. D., Van Veslor, E., & Ruderman, M. N. (2010). Introduction: Our viewpoint of leadership development. In E. Van Veslor, C. D. McCauley, & M. N. Ruderman (Eds.), *The center for creative leadership handbook of leadership development* (pp. 1–26). San Francisco, CA: Wiley.

McDowell-Larsen, S. (2012). *The care and feeding of the leader's brain.* White paper. Center for Creative Leadership, Greensboro, NC.

Medina, J. (2008). *Brain rules.* Seattle, WA: Pear Press.

Mehling, W. E., Wrubel, J., Daubenmier, J. J., Price, C. J., Kerr, C. E., Silow, J., ... Stewart, A. L. (2011). Body Awareness: A phenomenological inquiry into the common ground of mind-body therapies. *Philosophy, Ethics, and Humanities in Medicine, 6*(6). doi: 10.1186/1747-5341-6-6

Meurs, J. A., & Perrewé, P. L. (2011). Cognitive activation theory of stress: An integrative theoretical approach to work stress. *Journal of Management, 37*(4), 1043–1068.

Nolen-Hoeksema, S., & Morrow, J. (1991). A prospective study of depression and posttraumatic stress symptoms after a natural disaster: The 1989 Loma Prieta Earthquake. *Journal of Personality and Social Psychology, 61*(1), 115–121.

Nolen-Hoeksema, S., Wisco, B. E., & Lyubomirsky, S. (2008). Rethinking rumination. *Perspectives on Psychological Science, 3*(5), 400–424.

Owen, A. M., Hampshire, A., Grahn, J. A., Stenton, R., Dajani, S., Burns, A. S., ... Bullard, C. J. (2010). Putting brain training to the test. *Nature, 465*(June), 775–778.

Page, K., & Vella-Brodrick, D. (2009). The 'what', 'why' and 'how' of employee well-being: A new model. *Social Indicators Research, 90*(3), 441–458.

Pavlides, C., Nivón, L. G., & McEwen, B. S. (2002). Effects of chronic stress on hippocampal long-term potentiation. *Hippocampus, 12*(2), 245–257.

Quigg, A. M. (Ed.). (2015). *The handbook of dealing with workplace bullying.* Surrey: Ashgate Publishing, Ltd.

Ruderman, M. N., & Clerkin, C. (2015). Using mindfulness to improve high potential development. *Industrial and Organizational Psychology*, 8(04), 694−698.

Sapolsky, R. M. (2004). *Why zebras don't get ulcers: The acclaimed guide to stress, stress-related diseases, and coping*. London: Macmillan.

Sedlmeier, P., Eberth, J., Schwarz, M., Zimmermann, D., Haarig, F., Jaeger, S., & Kunze, S. (2012). The psychological effects of meditation: A meta-analysis. *Psychological Bulletin*, 138(6), 1139−1171.

Siegel, D. J. (2012). *Pocket guide to interpersonal neurobiology: An integrative handbook of the Mind (Norton Series on Interpersonal Neurobiology)*. New York, NY: WW Norton & Company.

Syrek, C. J., & Antoni, C. H. (2014). Unfinished tasks foster rumination and impair sleeping — Particularly if leaders have high performance expectations. *Journal of Occupational Health Psychology*, 19(4), 490−499. doi:10.1037/a0037127.

Tamim, H., Castel, E. S., Jamnik, V., Keir, P. J., Grace, S. L., Gledhill, N., & Macpherson, A. K. (2009). Tai Chi workplace program for improving musculoskeletal fitness among female computer users. *Work*, 34(3), 331−338.

Umberson, D., & Montez, J. K. (2010). Social relationships and health a flashpoint for health policy. *Journal of Health and Social Behavior*, 51(1), 54−66.

Viswesvaran, C., Sanchez, J. I., & Fisher, J. (1999). The role of social support in the process of work stress: A meta-analysis. *Journal of Vocational Behavior*, 54(2), 314−334.

Walker, M. P., Stickgold, R., Alsop, D., Gaab, N., & Schlaug, G. (2005). Sleep-dependent motor memory plasticity in the human brain. *Neuroscience*, 133(4), 911−917.

Wang, C., Bannuru, R., Ramel, J., Kupelnick, B., Scott, T., & Schmid, C. H. (2010). Tai Chi on psychological well-being: Systematic review and meta-analysis. *BMC Complementary and Alternative Medicine*, 10(1). doi: 10.1186/1472-6882-10-23

Wayne, S. J., Shore, L. M., & Liden, R. C. (1997). Perceived organizational support and leader-member exchange: A social exchange perspective. *Academy of Management Journal*, 40(1), 82−111.

Williamson, A. M., & Feyer, A. M. (2000). Moderate sleep deprivation produces impairments in cognitive and motor performance equivalent to legally prescribed levels of alcohol intoxication. *Occupational and Environmental Medicine*, 57(10), 649−655.

Wilson, B., Mickes, L., Stolarz-Fantino, S., Evrard, M., & Fantino, E. (2015). Increased false-memory susceptibility after mindfulness meditation. *Psychological Science*, 26(10), 1567−1573.

Wood, A. M., Froh, J. J., & Geraghty, A. W. (2010). Gratitude and well-being: A review and theoretical integration. *Clinical Psychology Review*, 30, 890−905.

Yancey, A. K., McCarthy, W. J., Taylor, W. C., Merlo, A., Gewa, C., Weber, M. D., & Fielding, J. E. (2004). The Los Angeles lift off: A sociocultural environmental change intervention to integrate physical activity into the workplace. *Preventive Medicine*, 38(6), 848−856.

Youssef, C. M., & Luthans, F. (2007). Positive organizational behavior in the workplace the impact of hope, optimism, and resilience. *Journal of Management*, 33(5), 774−800.

Zawadzka, A. M., & Szabowska-Walaszczyk, A. (2014). Does self-improvement explain well-being in life and at workplace? Analysis based on selected measures of well-being. *Polish Psychological Bulletin*, 45(2), 134−141.

# ABOUT THE AUTHORS AND EDITORS

## GUEST EDITORS

**Cathleen Clerkin,** Ph.D., is Research Faculty member at the Center for Creative Leadership. She is an interdisciplinary researcher whose areas of expertise include women's leadership, social identity management, holistic leadership development, and creativity and innovation. Prior to joining CCL, Cathleen led a number of research initiatives both in the USA and overseas and has won multiple awards and honors for her research, including recognition from the National Science Foundation. Cathleen graduated Phi Beta Kappa from the University of California, Berkeley, and earned her M.S. and Ph.D. degrees in psychology from the University of Michigan, Ann Arbor. She completed a post-doctoral fellowship at the Center for Creative Leadership.

**William A. Gentry**, Ph.D. is currently the Director of Leadership Insights and Analytics and a Senior Research Scientist at the Center for Creative Leadership. He is also an adjunct assistant professor at Guilford College and an associate member of the graduate faculty at the University of North Carolina, Charlotte. Bill has more than 70 academic presentations, has been featured in more than 50 internet and newspaper outlets, and has published more than 40 articles on leadership and other topics in the fields of industrial-organizational psychology and organizational behavior. His book titled *Be the Boss Everyone Wants to Work For: A Guide for New Leaders* is now available.

## EDITORS

**Jonathon R. B. Halbesleben**, Ph.D., is the Associate Dean for Research and HealthSouth Chair of Health Care Management in Culverhouse College of Commerce at the University of Alabama. He received his Ph.D. in industrial/organizational psychology from the University of Oklahoma. His research concerning employee well-being and relationships in and out of

187

the workplace has been published in such journals as the *Journal of Applied Psychology, Journal of Management, Journal of Organizational Behavior, Journal of Occupational Health Psychology*, and *Leadership Quarterly*, among others. He is co-editor of *Research in Occupational Stress and Well-Being* and *Research in Personnel and Human Resources*. He serves of the editorial boards of the *Journal of Applied Psychology, Journal of Management, Organizational Behavior and Human Decision Processes, Journal of Business and Psychology*, and *Journal of Occupational Health Psychology*. He is a fellow of the American Psychological Society and Society for Industrial/Organizational Psychology, and is a member of the Academy of Management, Society of Occupational Health Psychology, and Society for Human Resource Management.

**Pamela L. Perrewé,** Ph.D. is the Haywood and Betty Taylor Eminent Scholar of Business Administration, Professor of Sport Management, and Distinguished Research Professor at Florida State University. Dr. Perrewé has focused her research interests in the areas of mentoring, job stress, coping, organizational politics, emotion and social influence. Dr. Perrewé has published over 40 books and book chapters and approximately 120 journal articles in journals such as *Academy of Management Journal, Journal of Management, Journal of Applied Psychology, Organizational Behavior and Human Decision Processes, Journal of Organizational Behavior, Journal of Occupational Health Psychology*, and *Personnel Psychology*. She has served as a member of the Editorial Review Board for *Academy of Management Journal, Journal of Occupational Health Psychology, Human Resource Management Review*, and *Leadership and Organizational Studies*. She has fellow status with Southern Management Association, the Society for Industrial and Organizational Psychology, Association for Psychological Science, and the American Psychological Association.

**Christopher C. Rosen,** Ph.D., is Professor in the Sam M. Walton College of Business at the University of Arkansas. He received a B.A. degree in Psychology and Economics from Washington and Lee University, his M.A. degree in Industrial/Organizational Psychology and Human Resource Management from Appalachian State University, and his Ph.D. in Industrial/Organizational Psychology from the University of Akron. His research broadly considers how work life experiences affect the well-being, attitudes, and performance of organizational members. Dr. Rosen's research has also focused on methodological questions pertaining to the measurement and modeling of psychological constructs. His research has appeared in outlets such as *Academy of Management Journal, Journal of*

*Applied Psychology, Journal of Management, Journal of Organizational Behavior, Organizational Behavior and Human Decision Processes, Organization Science,* and *Personnel Psychology.* He is currently on the editorial boards of *Group and Organization Management, Journal of Applied Psychology, Journal of Occupational and Organizational Psychology, Journal of Organizational Behavior, Journal of Management,* and *Organizational Behavior and Human Decision Processes.* In addition, Dr. Rosen is an associate editor for *Journal of Business and Psychology.*

# AUTHORS

**Melissa K. Carsten** is Associate Professor of Management at Winthrop University. Dr. Carsten's research interests are in the areas of organizational leadership and followership. Specifically, she studies followers' roles in the leadership process and how followers can help leaders advance organizational objectives. She has published articles in peer-reviewed journals such as *The Leadership Quarterly, Organizational Dynamics, Journal of Organizational Behavior,* and the *Journal of Occupational and Organizational Psychology.* She is also a member of the editorial board for *Group and Organization Management.* Dr. Carsten has received several best paper awards for her work on followership and published several edited books on the topic.

**Rachel Clapp-Smith** is Associate Professor of Leadership in the College of Business at Purdue University Calumet. She received her Ph.D. in Organizational Behavior and Leadership at the University of Nebraska and MBA in International Management at Thunderbird, the School of Global Management. Dr. Clapp-Smith has devoted her research to Global Mindset and Global Leadership Development, publishing articles in journals such as the *Journal of Leadership and Organizational Studies, Human Resource Management, Cross-Cultural Management, European Journal of International Management,* and the *Journal of Business Studies.* She has also published a chapter in *Global Mindset: Advances in International Management* and in a volume of *Advances in Global Leadership.* Dr. Clapp-Smith has presented at a number of annual meetings of the Academy of Management and International Leadership Association. She is a co-coordinator of the Network of Leadership Scholars and Director of The Leadership Center at Purdue University Calumet.

**Malissa A. Clark**, Ph.D., is Assistant Professor of Industrial-Organizational Psychology at the University of Georgia. She received her B.A. from the University of Michigan, and her M.A. and Ph.D. from Wayne State University. Her research interests center around work-family issues, workaholism, gender, and affective dynamics at work. Her research has been published in journals such as *Journal of Applied Psychology, Journal of Management*, and *Journal of Organizational Behavior*.

**Kristin L. Cullen-Lester**, Ph.D., is Senior Research Scientist at the Center for Creative Leadership (CCL®). She earned her M.S. and Ph.D. in industrial/organizational psychology from Auburn University. Her work focuses on improving leaders' understanding of organizational networks and the ability of organizations to facilitate collective leadership, complex collaboration, and change across organizational boundaries. Kristin's research has been published in the *Journal of Management, The Leadership Quarterly*, and *Journal of Vocational Behavior* among others. She recently co-guested edited a special issue of *The Leadership Quarterly* on Collective and Network Approaches to Leadership.

**Jennifer K. Dimoff**, M.Sc., is an advanced Ph.D. Candidate in Industrial/Organizational Psychology at Saint Mary's University in Nova Scotia, Canada, where she completed her Master's of Science degree in Applied Psychology. With a background in the biological sciences from Queen's University in Ontario, Canada, her research interests include biological markers of stress and psychological resilience, as well as leadership, employee mental health, and occupational health. As part of her graduate work, Jennifer developed the Mental Health Awareness Training (MHAT), one of the first scientifically evaluated mental health training programs for organizational leaders in Canada.

**Alexandra Gerbasi**, Ph.D., is Professor at the University of Surrey. Her research focuses on the effects of positive and negative ties within the workplace, and their effects on performance, well-being, thriving, affect and turnover. Her research has appeared *in Journal of Applied Psychology, Journal of Management, Social Psychology Quarterly, Journal of Strategic Information Systems, Organizational Dynamics*, and in several books. Her research has been supported by the National Science Foundation and Agence Nationale de la Recherche. She received her Ph.D. from Stanford University.

**Tracy L. Griggs** is an Assistant Professor in the Department of Management and Marketing at Winthrop University. She earned her Ph.D. in Industrial-Organizational Psychology from the University of Georgia.

Prior to joining the College of Business at Winthrop University, Dr. Griggs held appointments in the Department of Management at the University of North Carolina Asheville and the Department of Psychology at Winthrop University. She teaches courses in the areas of Human Resource Management and Organizational Behavior. Dr. Griggs' research focuses on employee career experiences including career development, career management, work-life balance, and leadership development.

**Michelle M. Hammond** works at the University of Limerick, Ireland, teaching Organisational Behaviour and Work Psychology. She earned her M.S. and Ph.D. in Industrial/Organizational Psychology from the Pennsylvania State University. Her research focuses on understanding the influence of leadership on employee well-being at work, including factors such as meaningful work, work-life balance, and creativity and innovation. Additionally her research seeks to understand the process of leadership development across multiple domains of life. She co-authored an award-winning book on leader development entitled *An Integrative Theory of Leader Development: Connecting Adult Development, Identity, and Expertise* and has published in academic journals including *Human Resource Management Review*, *Journal of Vocational Behavior*, and *Journal of Managerial Psychology*, among others. She is also the Course Director for the Masters in Work and Organisational Psychology/Behaviour and is a Registered Psychologist in Ireland.

**P. D. Harms** received his Ph.D. in Psychology from the University of Illinois at Urbana-Champaign in 2008. He is currently an Assistant Professor of Management at the University of Alabama. His research focuses on the assessment and development of personality, leadership, and psychological well-being. This work has been published in over 50 peer-reviewed articles and has been featured in popular media outlets such as CNN, Scientific American, Forbes, and the BBC. Dr. Harms is currently engaged in research partnerships with the U.S. Army, the U.S. Department of Labor, and the National Aeronautics and Space Administration (NASA).

**E. Kevin Kelloway** is the Tier 1 Canada Research Chair in Occupational Health Psychology and Professor of Psychology at Saint Mary's University, Halifax, NS. A graduate of Queen's University, his research interests include leadership, occupational health and safety, workplace violence and occupational stress. A prolific researcher, he is the author/editor of 15 books and over 150 articles and chapters. He has been elected a Fellow of the Association for Psychological Science, the Canadian

Psychological Association, the International Association of Applied Psychology and the Society for Industrial/Organizational Psychology. He is Associate Editor of *Work & Stress* and the *Journal of Occupational Health Psychology*, the *Journal of Organizational Effectiveness: People and Performance* and is Section Editor (Conceptual Reviews) of *Stress & Health*. He currently serves as the President of the Canadian Psychological Association – Canada's national association for psychology.

**Gretchen Vogelgesang Lester** is Assistant Professor at San Jose State University. She teaches the capstone strategic management course, as well as a global leadership course located in Silicon Valley. She earned her Ph. D. from the University of Nebraska – Lincoln and her MBA from DePaul University. Her research encompasses global leadership development as well as transparent communication between leaders and followers. She has published in such journals as *The Leadership Quarterly*, the *Academy of Management Learning and Education*, the *Journal of Leadership and Organization Studies*, the *Canadian Journal of Administrative Sciences*, and *Human Resource Development Review*. She also has presented her work at the Academy of Management Conferences and serves as a reviewer for a number of leadership journals.

**Jesse S. Michel**, Ph.D., is Assistant Professor in the Department of Psychology at Auburn University. His current research activities revolve around the dynamics between work-family domains (e.g., work-family conflict, work-family balance, benefits of multiple life roles), the role of personality and individual differences in the workplace, and scale development and validation projects. His research has appeared in journals such as *Journal of Organizational Behavior*, *Journal of Vocational Behavior*, and *Journal of Business and Psychology*.

**Michael E. Palanski** is Associate Professor of Management at the Saunders College of Business at the Rochester Institute of Technology in Rochester, NY. He teaches undergraduate, graduate, and executive MBA classes in leadership, organizational behavior, and business ethics. He also teaches leadership skills development and conducts leadership coaching in RIT's online executive MBA program. He has published numerous peer-reviewed articles in journals such as *The Leadership Quarterly*, *Journal of Business Ethics*, and *Journal of Management Education*, and is a noted expert on leader integrity. He holds a Ph.D. in Organizational Behavior/Leadership from SUNY Binghamton, an MA in Theology from Covenant Theological Seminary, and a BS from Grove City College. Prior to joining academia, he worked as a retail product manager for a Fortune 500 company and as an online banking specialist.

**Marian N. Ruderman** is currently a Senior Fellow and Director, Research Horizons at the Creative Leadership (CCL®). Marian has written several books and assessments including Standing at the Crossroads: Next Steps for High-Achieving Women and the WorkLife Indicator. Her research has been published in such journals as the *Journal of Applied Psychology* and the *Academy of Management Journal*. She holds a B.A. from Cornell University and a M.A. and a Ph.D. in Organizational Psychology from the University of Michigan. Marian is a Fellow of the Society for Industrial and Organizational Psychology (SIOP) and the American Psychological Association (APA).

**Seth M. Spain** received his Ph.D. in Industrial and Organizational Psychology from the University of Illinois at Urbana-Champaign. He is currently an Assistant Professor of Organizational Behavior and leadership and fellow of the Center for Leadership Studies at Binghamton University. His research focuses on personality, individual job performance, and leadership. His research has been featured by the *Wall Street Journal*, *Time*, and *CNN*. He has appeared on CBS This Morning and National Public Radio to discuss his research.

**Gregory W. Stevens**, Ph.D., is Research Analyst with Globoforce. He received his Ph.D. and M.A. in Industrial-Organizational Psychology from Auburn University. His research interests include employee recognition, work investment, organizational change management, and employee well-being. He is a member of the Society for Industrial and Organizational Psychology and has been published in such journals as the *Journal of Applied Behavioral Science, Human Resource Development Review, Advances in Healthcare Management, Stress and Health*, and *Journal of Business Ethics*.

**Mary Uhl-Bien** is the BNSF Endowed Professor of Leadership in the Neeley School of Business at Texas Christian University (TCU). She has been a Visiting Scholar in Australia, Sweden, Portugal and Spain. Mary's research focuses on complexity leadership, relational leadership, and followership, and has appeared in such journals as *Academy of Management Journal, Journal of Applied Psychology, Journal of Management*, and *The Leadership Quarterly*. Her papers on complexity leadership theory and followership theory have been recognized with best paper awards, and she is senior editor of the Leadership Horizons series for Information Age Publishing.

**Sean White** is a Ph.D. student at Grenoble Ecole de Management. His research focus is Entrepreneurship and Social Networks, observing the support provided to entrepreneurs through their direct and indirect relationships. He holds a bachelor's degree in Psychology from Universidade Presbiteriana Mackenzie and a Master's degree from Insper. He was a career counselor and clinical psychologist prior to joining the Ph. D. program.

**Dustin Wood** received his Ph.D. in Psychology from the University of Illinois at Urbana-Champaign in 2007. He is currently a Research Fellow at the Department of Management at the University of Alabama. He has authored over 40 peer-reviewed articles in theoretical and empirical journals on topics related to the measurement of personality-related characteristics, and modeling how they influence one another and the environment over time.

**Lauren Zimmerman** is currently a Senior Analyst on Johnson & Johnson's Organizational Analytics team. Concurrently, she's completing her Ph.D. at the University of Georgia, where she obtained her M.S. in Industrial-Organizational Psychology in 2015. She received a B.S. in Psychology from High Point University in High Point, NC. Her core research interests include work-family issues, emotions within the workplace, workaholism, and women's experiences of opting-out and opting-in to the workforce.